NONVERBAL LEARNING DISABILITIES

Nonverbal
Learning Disabilities

Cesare Cornoldi
Irene C. Mammarella
Jodene Goldenring Fine

Foreword by Linda S. Siegel

THE GUILFORD PRESS
New York   London

The authors have checked with sources believed to be reliable in their efforts to
provide information that is complete and generally in accord with the standards
of practice that are accepted at the time of publication. However, in view of the
possibility of human error or changes in behavioral, mental health, or medical
sciences, neither the authors, nor the editors and publisher, nor any other party
who has been involved in the preparation or publication of this work warrants
that the information contained herein is in every respect accurate or complete,
and they are not responsible for any errors or omissions or the results obtained
from the use of such information. Readers are encouraged to confirm the
information contained in this book with other sources.

Library of Congress Cataloging-in-Publication Data

Names: Cornoldi, Cesare, author. | Mammarella, Irene C., author. | Fine,
    Jodene Goldenring.
Title: Nonverbal learning disabilities / Cesare Cornoldi, Irene C.
    Mammarella, Jodene Goldenring Fine.
Description: New York: The Guilford Press, [2016] | Includes bibliographical
    references and index.
Identifiers: LCCN 2016029302 | ISBN 9781462527588 (hardback)
Subjects: LCSH: Nonverbal learning disabilities. | Learning disabled
    children. | Social skills in children. | BISAC: PSYCHOLOGY /
    Neuropsychology. | MEDICAL / Neuroscience. | EDUCATION / Special
    Education / Learning Disabilities. | SOCIAL SCIENCE / Social Work. |
    PSYCHOLOGY / Developmental / Child.
Classification: LCC RJ506.L4 C66 2016 | DDC 618.92/86889—dc23
LC record available at *https://lccn.loc.gov/2016029302*

About the Authors

Cesare Cornoldi is Full Professor in the Department of General Psychology at the University of Padua, Italy, where he also manages a laboratory that provides assessment and intervention for learning disabilities and developmental disorders. He conducts research both nationally and internationally on memory, mental imagery, learning disabilities, and human intelligence. Dr. Cornoldi serves on the editorial boards of many national and international journals and has been visiting professor at a number of universities, including Columbia University, New York University, and the University of California, Irvine. He has served as president of the European Society for Cognitive Psychology, among other associations, and is a Fellow of the International Academy for Research in Learning Disabilities and the Association for Psychological Science. His publications include 300 peer-reviewed journal articles, 10 books, and numerous widely used Italian achievement tests.

Irene C. Mammarella, PhD, is Lecturer in the Department of Developmental and Social Psychology at the University of Padua, Italy, where she directs a postgraduate course in Developmental Psychopathology. She conducts clinical practice at the laboratory directed by Cesare Cornoldi. Her main areas of research are nonverbal learning disability, mathematical learning disability, the role of working memory in both academic achievement and calculation, and visuospatial abilities in high-functioning autism. The author of many peer-reviewed journal articles, Dr. Mammarella serves on the editorial board of the *Journal of Experimental Child Psychology.*

Jodene Goldenring Fine, PhD, is Associate Professor of School Psychology at Michigan State University, where she teaches graduate students and conducts research on autism, nonverbal learning disability, and dyslexia, using neuropsychological and neuroimaging techniques. Dr. Fine has lectured worldwide on the importance of a neuropsychological perspective in education, particularly with regard to the identification and treatment of children with learning challenges. A member of the National Academy of Neuropsychology and the International Academy for Research in Learning Disabilities, she served on the editorial board of *Psychological Assessment.*

Foreword

Those of us who work as researchers and/or clinicians with people with specific learning disabilities have long been aware of a problem called "nonverbal learning disability" (NLD). This disability is a subtle one. Dealing with an NLD is like trying to capture a soap bubble floating in the air; just when you think you are next to it and ready to burst it, it disappears before you can grasp it. And just when you think you understand NLD, an individual appears who does not fit the entire pattern but has some of the characteristics.

While keeping in mind the complexities of and individual differences among the brains and behaviors of individuals with learning difficulties, the authors have identified the major characteristics of an NLD. The deficits in social perceptions and social behavior at the core of this disability are well documented in this book. There is evidence of deficits in perceiving facial expressions and gestures. The prosody or voice modulation of a child with an NLD is often not quite correct. Problems with developing social relationships and finding friends are pervasive characteristics.

Cognitive and motor difficulties are also present. Trouble with handwriting and copying writing from paper or the blackboard, and problems with fine-motor coordination, affect most of the people with NLD. A possible defining characteristic, although the evidence is not conclusive, is difficulties with two- and three-dimensional visuospatial concepts. Problems with mathematics, especially calculation, are often present. Decoding difficulties are usually not present and reading comprehension is usually fine, but may deteriorate under timed conditions.

Typically, the oral language skills and the ability to tell imaginative stories are present in individuals with NLD but not evident in their written work. In assessing people for NLD, it is important to search beyond their written productions and examine their oral language skills.

Cesare Cornoldi, Irene C. Mammarella, and Jodene Goldenring Fine are aware of the definitional problems regarding an NLD and the complexities of attempting to understand the nature of it. They have advanced the field by a comprehensive and integrative review of the literature and have captured the major difficulties of people who have this problem. Perhaps the best approach is not to fit everybody into a single definition but to consider subtypes with partially overlapping characteristics.

One of the values of this book is that the authors examine research results in more than group means. They advocate studying individual variation and individual differences. They use case studies to aid in the understanding of the complexities of this learning problem. This approach can be quite productive and can help us understand the value and limits of NLD as a diagnostic category. If some portion of the individuals with NLD do not show a particular pattern, then it is possible that there are subtypes within this population, an issue that it is worth considering.

Although the literature on intervention is scarce, the authors review that literature and provide worthwhile suggestions. A particularly important feature is that they advocate dealing with the family, not just the child with an NLD.

There is also an attempt to differentiate NLD from high-functioning autism and to present research to help clarify the distinction. This issue is significant for the field.

This book is an important step forward. As the ancient Chinese philosopher Lao Tzu noted, "A journey of a thousand miles begins with a single step." The authors have bravely ventured into new territory. There will doubtless be disagreements and missteps, but this book represents an important step forward.

LINDA S. SIEGEL, PhD
University of British Columbia

Preface

The initial idea for this book emerged following an international symposium on nonverbal learning disabilities (NLD) held in Padua, Italy. Embraced by the historical rooms frequented by Nicolaus Copernicus, Giovanni Morgagni, Galileo Galilei, and many other distinguished scholars who once resided within the University of Padua, we found ourselves deep in conversation regarding how best to characterize children with NLD more than 800 years after the university was established. We were attending the International Academy for Research in Learning Disabilities (IARLD) annual convention, which brings together researchers from 30 countries around the world. Our symposium included several experts on NLD: John M. Davis, Jessica Broitman, Kenneth Adams, and Bonny Forrest. Our common interests brought us together for a traditional meal in a charming downtown old "trattoria," where we shared many ideas and intentions. We all agreed that an effort to organize and unify knowledge on NLD and to develop a broad perspective was necessary from both a scientific and a clinical point of view.

Decidedly lacking in modern times, a coherent, unified description of the NLD profile is critical for developing sound systematic analyses for researchers of NLD. Additionally, more clinical clarity for diagnostic assessment and empirically tested interventions is needed to guide practitioners. Such a systematic approach would address the current paradoxical situation whereby a large majority of clinicians working with neurodevelopmental disorders recognize the syndrome of NLD but the clinical specification for NLD remains vague or even questionable. Thus, a major impetus for the book is that despite the lack of a full consensus, the diagnosis of NLD is rather frequent, either alone or in association with other formally recognized diagnoses. This situation can only be improved with the introduction of well-identified criteria.

The present book represents a progressive maturation of knowledge based on research, discussion, and collaboration among researchers and clinicians from various countries around the world. It attempts to unify and formalize the many common ideas in the field of NLD that have accompanied our work for many years. The book is organized in eight chapters. Chapter 1 provides an in-depth historical background on NLD. We illustrate how the field started and found traction in the pioneering work of Helmer Myklebust, Doris Johnson, and Byron Rourke. The chapter lays out both the origin and the challenges inherent in the label of NLD and provides a rationale for an updated synthesis of the field.

Chapter 2 reviews the cognitive and academic weaknesses and strengths of children with NLD. In particular, we evaluate evidence concerning visual perception, motor coordination, visuoconstruction, spatial abilities, language, visuospatial working memory, mental imagery, executive functions, long-term memory, and reasoning. Researchers have used slightly different populations, so we offer a table that helps the reader recognize the research methods and sample sources for the studies. A similar table is presented for research on academic learning difficulties, where reading, decoding, and spelling are consistently seen as strengths, but there is variation on reading comprehension, handwriting, calculation, and other mathematics aspects. Chapter 3 similarly reviews evidence concerning emotional and social difficulties of children with NLD with particular reference to social cue encoding and interpretation, attention, social functioning, and psychological adjustment.

NLD appears to be a neurodevelopmental disorder with genetic influences and early indicators, so Chapter 4 presents neurological and anatomical evidence found to date. Because of the small amount of neurobiological research conducted on NLD thus far, the chapter also presents a historical perspective.

Early work on the biological bases of learning disabilities in general and of NLD that initiated the old label of "right-hemisphere learning disability" is discussed. Then recent studies are presented illustrating the role of better-defined neurological structures, including the hypothesis the smaller splenium of the corpus callosum may play a critical role.

Chapter 5 utilizes a systematic overview of literature and clinical reports to synthesize a proposal for diagnostic criteria that could form the basis for both research and clinical recognition of NLD. The criteria outlined are consistent with current diagnostic methods, such as the fifth edition of the *Diagnostic and Statistical Manual of Mental Disorders*. We view consistency in diagnosis as critical to moving the field forward in terms of both research and clinical practice.

Assessment issues are the subject of Chapter 6. We examine assessment from the practitioner's point of view, discussing important issues for differential diagnosis. Interviews, questionnaires, and standardized tests recommended for NLD are presented with particular attention to the most useful procedures. Most importantly, we take an international perspective, considering the experiences collected not only in the historically dominant-for-the-field North America but also in European countries. Specific procedures not easily available to the practitioner are described and also included.

Chapter 7 illustrates intervention strategies. We begin with a review of the small body of existing literature followed by a presentation of general guidelines. Policies and procedures appropriate to supporting children with NLD in school, family, and community settings are presented. Finally, we suggest approaches that might be taken for psychological intervention. Included in our discussion are general guidelines for clinical intervention with the child with NLD, noting that this involves systematic planning, accurate assessment, establishment of priorities for intervention, and use of a multimodal approach to intervention that considers the child, the school, the family, and social contexts. Ideas for supporting cognitive, psychological, academic, communicative, and executive skills are presented.

To better illustrate our thoughts on assessment and intervention, Chapter 8 presents three case studies. These cases are taken from clinical evaluations and interventions provided to children (of various ages) in the United States and in Europe. Specific diagnostic procedures and instruments are discussed along with thoughts regarding rehabilitation for the children.

In summary, we have tried to offer an updated overview of the field of NLD that is as complete as can be, given the current state of the science and clinical wisdom. At the same time, we have considered the needs of both the researcher and the clinician, offering a systematic, consultable, and readable review not only of research evidence but also of good practices. We hope our readers will appreciate and share our deep interest in NLD. We further hope that our readers use our work to serve this fascinating and underserved population.

Contents

CHAPTER ONE

Past and Present Research

The Nonverbal Learning Disability Profile

Imagine a child with an average overall IQ, a good vocabulary, who can read and speak well, but has difficulties in written calculation and poor handwriting that is characterized by uneven and different-sized letters. In addition, this hypothetical child can appear uncoordinated when performing athletic activities, may have difficulties in drawing and in completing simple visuo-spatial tasks such as puzzles, and may show a poor sense of direction. Some additional problems may be observed, for example, in judging facial expressions or nonverbal communication. This child presents with at least average intelligence and commensurate verbal skills, but a series of symptoms specific to non-language-based domains are present. A descriptive category, *specific nonverbal disorder,* also called "nonverbal learning disability" (NLD), has been used by clinicians and researchers alike, which directly contrasts to *specific language disorder.* The NLD category captures an array of characteristics rather than focusing on a single symptom—for example, motor coordination as in the case of developmental coordination disorder (DCD), which requires a dramatic weakness in this aspect (i.e., below 1.5 or 2 standard deviations). It is worth noting that this is not necessarily the case of children with NLD, and at the same time NLD presents a series of weaknesses that are not present in the case of DCD.

1

Children like the one described above have always existed as is demonstrated by the description of some famous people from the past. In a brilliant book, Siegel (2013, pp. 64–68) describes the case of the Danish writer and poet Hans Christian Andersen using these words: "He had difficulties reading maps and memorizing material. He describes himself as being overpowered by grammar, geography, and mathematics. Hans Christian Andersen lived in a dream world. He was a loner who rarely played with other boys. He had difficulty with social skills and described himself as friendless." Siegel concluded that Andersen had NLD. Another example of a possible case of NLD can be found in *The Tongue Set Free*; the autobiography of Elias Canetti (who won the Nobel Prize for literature) in which he describes his difficulties: "There is nothing healthier for a child who learns easily than utter failure in some field or other. I was the worst in drawing" (1979, p. 227); and in another passage: "When I brought home natural-science booklets from school, copying the pictures assiduously—a real strain on a bad draughtsman—she pushed me away; I could never get her interested in them" (p. 171).

The general impression is that children with NLD characteristics may be rather numerous. For example, making reference to the critical feature of low visuospatial intelligence in combination with average to high verbal intelligence, it can be argued that the number of children presenting this aspect corresponds to the number of children having the opposite profile (i.e., a low verbal compared with a high visuospatial intelligence). However, the NLD profile has not received the same interest as has specific language disorder. The modest attention to NLD may be attributed to at least two main reasons. First, in the past the school systems of many countries focused on verbal skills and instructional verbal materials, including textbooks and oral lessons. Therefore, children presenting verbal problems were awarded more intense attention by teachers. In contrast, traditional teachers showed less concern for a child failing in nonverbal activities such as drawing, athletic skill, or nonverbal communication. Second, the NLD profile presents some overlap (see Figure 1.1) with other clinical profiles like autism spectrum disorder (ASD), dysgraphia, dyscalculia, DCD, attention-deficit/hyperactivity disorder (ADHD), depression, social anxiety, and pragmatic communication disorder, and, given the greater popularity of these

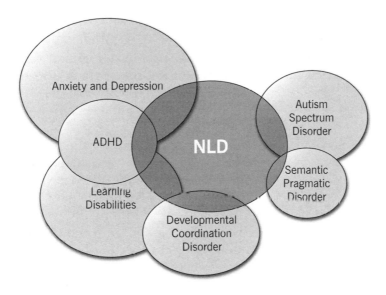

FIGURE 1.1. An example of profiles partly overlapping with NLD.

profiles, may be confounded with them. Children with NLD may receive one or more of those diagnoses. However, none of them quite captures the overall pattern of the NLD profile. In addition, there are examples of children with a diagnosis of NLD who do not present weaknesses in any of the dimensions covered by the other diagnoses (see, e.g., Forrest, 2004).

It is possible that, for these reasons, an extensive description of NLD has been given only relatively recently, in the second half of the 20th century. The relatively recent scientific description does not mean that the profile of NLD is unimportant. In fact, a similar story could be written about the historical acceptance of the diagnosis of ASD. Similarly, learning disabilities (LD) in general were described before the 20th century but were studied in depth only after 1960.

The Origins of Research on LD

Interest in LD, and in particular in dyslexia, began at the end of 19th century, when school became mandatory in most countries and the interest in children with learning difficulties increased.

In particular, in 1881 in Germany, Oswald Berkhan offered the description of a child with severe reading difficulties and a few years later the ophthalmologist Rudolf Berlin coined the term "dyslexia" (Pagel, 1901). During the same years in the United Kingdom, James Hinshelwood and William Pringle Morgan described cases with normal intelligence and vision but blind to written words (Snowling, 1996).

At that time, an emerging issue concerning the relationship between intelligence and reading led, some years later, to Alfred Binet and Theodore Simon's (Binet & Simon, 1948) development of the first intelligence test designed to identify children unable to follow normal school education. Additionally, the instrument led to interest in distinguishing children who, despite low achievement, had high intelligence. In the first half of the 20th century, researchers and clinicians focused on the inability to read and write, so studies were conducted on methods of treatment (see Orton, 1937).

During the first half of the 20th century, diagnostic and intervention procedures were not only devoted to reading and writing but also to nonverbal skills. For example, in Italy, Maria Montessori (1934) insisted on the relevance of sensory and nonverbal stimulation. In North America, around midcentury, Alfred Strauss and Laura Lehtinen (1947) published their classic book *Psychopathology and Education of the Brain-Injured Child,* illustrating cognitive deficits that could result in specific disorders, including perceptual and attentional deficits. Since that time, experts like Newell Kephart (1960), William Cruickshank and Daniel Hallahan (1961), Samuel Kirk and Winifred Kirk (1971), and Marianne Frostig and Phyllis Maslow (1973) proposed intervention programs for language, perceptual, and motor skills, while highlighting the influence of these cognitive processes on reading, handwriting, and calculation difficulties. Simultaneously, interest in nonverbal abilities increased in Europe. In 1951, René Zazzo edited a volume of the journal *Enfance* concerning dyslexia, which also included papers on nonverbal interventions, such as spatial organization (Galifret-Granjon, 1951) and rhythm (Stambak, 1951).

In European countries, special classrooms for children with general cognitive impairments were initiated wherein adjustments to the curriculum to meet the student's level of impairment were made, while the academic community moved toward a formal recognition of specific LD. According to Donald D. Hammill (1990), the first definition of LD was proposed by Samuel Kirk in 1962 (see Hammill, 1990) and was publicly presented during the first meeting of the Association for Children with Learning Disabilities (ACLD) in Chicago (1963). Six years later the National Advisory Committee on Handicapped Children published the first definition of LD and, in the same year, created the most important journal in the field: the *Journal of Learning Disabilities*. In the United States, a law protecting children with an LD (the Children with Specific Learning Disabilities Act 1970; Public Law 91-230) was established, fully recognizing the responsibility of the government to provide special instructional modifications.

Eventually, interest in LD moved toward finding specific cognitive and behavioral profiles in order to provide more targeted intervention. However, the focus was on the relationship between language difficulties and LD. In particular, attention was given to linguistic deficits as precursors of LD or as the verbal deficits underlying LD. An example of this clinical orientation toward verbal deficits and visuospatial strengths in LD is represented by the work of James Inglis and James S. Lawson (1987; Lawson & Inglis, 1985), involving more than 9,000 previously diagnosed cases. In a review of published data from the Wechsler Intelligence Scale for Children—Revised (WISC-R) and the Wechsler Intelligence Scale for Children (WISC; Wechsler, 1974) for children with LD, Lawson and Inglis (1985) found that the severity of deficits shown by children with LD in the WISC subtests was proportional to the degree of verbal content. On this basis they proposed an LD index that was directly related to performance in verbal subtests and inversely related to performance in nonverbal subtests.

Doris J. Johnson and Helmer R. Myklebust

As early as the 1960s, however, attention to a nonverbal subtype of LD was present in the insightful work of Johnson and Myklebust (Myklebust, 1975; Johnson & Myklebust, 1967; Boshes & Myklebust, 1964), who proposed a form of NLD. These scholars described children who had no serious language and reading problems, but had "persistent problems in right–left orientation, constructional tasks and arithmetic, whose deficit is not verbal, not academic in the usual sense, but who is unable to comprehend the significance of many aspects of his environment" (Johnson & Myklebust, 1967, p. 272).

The earliest description of NLD and the term "nonverbal learning disabilities" are attributed to these seminal researchers, who suggested that these children had difficulty in nonverbal aspects of their environment, while their verbal intelligence was at or above average. In their analysis, Johnson and Myklebust (1967) tried to define the characteristics of these children, focusing particularly on some nonverbal learning domains that could lead to selective deficits: (1) *perception,* meaning the ability to encode the whole and its salient parts of a configuration and to learn through pictures; (2) *processing of gestures,* or giving meaning to visual movements; (3) *motor learning,* the ability to learn motor patterns, such as those required in handwriting or using objects such as scissors; (4) *body image,* visualization of one's own body, associated with digital agnosia; (5) *spatial orientation,* the ability to establish a spatial relationship of the body with other objects, and to recall spatial locations; and (6) *left–right orientation,* laterality delay. Johnson and Myklebust also associated these dysfunctions with a syndrome described by Josef Gerstmann (see 1940) in the first half of the 20th century and characterized by problems in left–right orientation, digital agnosia, dyscalculia, and dysgraphia associated with a left-hemisphere parietal dysfunction.

Johnson and Myklebust (1967) also hypothesized two additional nonverbal domains that could reveal a disordered acquisition: *social perception,* for example, the ability to adapt and to anticipate the consequences of one's own behavior in response to socially relevant information; and the *regulation of attention/ monitoring systems,* or the child's ability to "scan, select, and hold internal events in a manner consistent with his circumstances" (p. 300). This work laid the foundation for the next wave of research, conducted by Byron P. Rourke.

Byron P. Rourke

The Myklebust proposal received some attention, but soon the field in this area was influenced by the work carried out by

Canadian neuropsychologist Byron P. Rourke. In his 40 years of research Rourke was very active, publishing a long series of studies, as well as developing a model explaining the typical deficits of children with NLD. The model proposed by Rourke soon differed from the description offered by Johnson and Myklebust, as reported by Johnson (personal communication, 2014).

Rourke spent his entire life studying and treating children with NLD as demonstrated by his interest in talking about NLD even a few days before his death (August 10, 2011). In a personal e-mail communication to Cesare Cornoldi, he tried to clear up some confusion in the current literature about the following question: Are deficits in visuospatial skills the primary cause of psychosocial disturbances in persons with NLD? His response was negative, because in his NLD model, "although deficits in visual–spatial–organizational skills are seen as a primary causal factor in the developmental emergence of psychosocial dysfunction in persons with NLD, these are characterized as only one of four sets of deficits that constitute the principal etiological bases for eventual psychosocial dysfunction." He concluded the communication with "Please let me know if there are any questions that you think I should add in my website," demonstrating his interest in disseminating knowledge on NLD (personal communication to Cesare Cornoldi). As already mentioned, Byron P. Rourke created and took care of his website, which is, unfortunately, no longer online, in which he summarized his NLD model and his research. We can divide Rourke's research into three periods: the first, during which he started studying NLD; the second, during which he developed an NLD model specifying a pattern of relative *assets* and *deficits* for describing the features of children with NLD; and a third period, during which he interpreted NLD as a unitary entity, referring to it as an NLD "syndrome."

In their first studies Rourke and collaborators (Rourke, 1985; Rourke & Finlayson, 1978; Rourke & Gates, 1981; Strang & Rourke, 1985) searched for subtypes of LD by attempting to isolate learners who are arithmetic disabled. In particular, Rourke and Finlayson (1978) selected three groups: (1) children with reading, spelling, and arithmetic impairments; (2) children who were relatively adept at arithmetic as compared with their performance in reading and spelling; and (3) an NLD group of children whose reading and spelling were average or above, but whose arithmetic performance was relatively deficient. By using a series of cognitive tests, they found that groups 1 and 2 were superior to group 3 on visuospatial abilities, while group 3 performed better than groups 1 and 2 on measures of verbal and auditory–perceptual abilities.

On the basis of his first period of research on NLD, in successive years Rourke developed his NLD model. According to Rourke (1989, 1995) NLD is characterized by deficits grouped into three main areas: neuropsychological, academic, and social–emotional/adaptational. Neuropsychological deficits include difficulties with tactile and visual perception, psychomotor coordination, tactile and visual attention, visuospatial memory, reasoning, verbosity, and lack of prosody. Academic deficits involve difficulties with math calculations, mathematical reasoning, reading comprehension, specific aspects of written language, and handwriting. Finally, social deficits include problems with social perception and social interaction. Rourke's (1995) model speculates that primary neuropsychological deficits lead to secondary deficits, which then lead to tertiary deficits, and so on. Primary neuropsychological deficits include tactile, visual perception, and motor coordination. In turn, secondary deficits (i.e., tactile and visual attention) lead to tertiary deficits, particularly in visuospatial memory, abstract reasoning, and specific aspects of speech and language. Specific, measurable impairments in academic performance, social functioning, and emotional well-being were considered to be direct by-products of this constellation of primary, secondary, and tertiary neuropsychological deficits.

During the third period of his research, Rourke not only better established the profile of NLD but also advanced some hypotheses on the neurological correlates of NLD. He started to examine the presence of an NLD profile in different disorders using the term "nonverbal syndrome" as an "umbrella" under which different problems and pathologies could be included.

The NLD Profile Associated with Other Disorders

Rourke's hypothetical NLD model proposed that hemispheric differential organization in white matter, both within and between hemispheres, as well as connectivity and the ratio of white to gray matter underlay the NLD symptoms. This "white-matter" model (Rourke, 1995) presumed that the deficits observed in NLD syndrome result from disturbances in the myelination of the extensive fiber tracts that constitute right-hemisphere anatomy. The hypothesis was then extended to a wide variety of congenital as well as acquired conditions. In addition, Rourke tried to extend the NLD clinical profile to at least three different situations: (1) cases with other diagnoses, such as Asperger syndrome (AS), velocardiofacial syndrome (22q11 deletion), Turner syndrome, and agenesis of the corpus callosum, who also have a nonverbal deficit profile; (2) cases with a specific nonverbal disorder who do not have severe academic difficulties; and (3) cases with a specific nonverbal disorder who also have severe learning problems. Rourke and coauthors additionally observed that the pattern of deficits in children with NLD appeared to change over time with changing demands at school and at home (Casey, Rourke, & Picard, 1991; Ozols & Rourke, 1991; Rourke, 1989, 1995). Table 1.1 summarizes the neurological diseases, disorders, and dysfunctions in which some characteristics of NLD could be observed, according to Rourke (2000).

Table 1.1, at level 1, lists the disorders in which all the assets and deficits of NLD can be manifest; at level 2 the majority of assets and deficits can be observed; with fairly clear evidence of NLD many of the assets and deficits are present (Rourke, 2000). It must be noted that Rourke mainly focused on medical illnesses, but also mentioned the case of neural dysfunctions. Notably, the white-matter model has met with some criticism (see Spreen, 2011; Fine, Semrud-Clikeman, Bledsoe, & Musielak, 2013, for critical reviews), although it remains the most comprehensively articulated model thus far. However, other authors (see, e.g., Stiles, Appelbaum, Nass, & Trauner, 2008; Vicari, Caravale, Carlesimo, Casadei, & Allemand, 2004) have specifically studied the effect of brain lesions on visuospatial skills without referring to them as an NLD syndrome. Still others have focused on brain functioning, and in particular on right-hemisphere activity, introducing the term "right-hemisphere disorder" (see, e.g., Voeller, 1986; Tranel, Hall, Olson, & Tranel, 1987).

TABLE 1.1. Neurological Diseases, Syndromes, and Dysfunctions in Which It Is Possible to Observe the NLD Profile

Level 1

- Callosal agenesis
- Asperger syndrome
- Velocardiofacial syndrome
- Williams syndrome
- de Lange syndrome
- Early hydrocephalus
- Turner syndrome
- Significant damage or dysfunction of the right cerebral hemisphere

Level 2

- Sotos syndrome
- Prophylactic treatment of some form of cancer affecting the brain
- Metachromatic leukodystrophy
- Congenital hypothyroidism
- Fetal alcohol syndrome

Fairly clear evidence of NLD

- Multiple sclerosis
- Traumatic brain injury
- Toxicant-induced encephalopathy and teratology
- Children with HIV and white matter disease
- Fragile X syndrome (high functioning)
- Triple X syndrome
- Leukodystrophy other than metachromatic
- Haemophilus influenzae meningitis
- Early-treated phenylketonuria
- Intraventricular hemorrhage
- Children with very low birth weight
- Congenital adrenal hyperplasia
- Insulin-dependent diabetes mellitus
- Fahr syndrome

Note. Based on Rourke (2000).

Right-Hemisphere LD

Among the different labels that have been used in an effort to define children with NLD appropriately—for example, *nonverbal disorders of learning* (Myklebust, 1975), *nonverbal learning syndrome* (Rourke, 1989, 1995), and *visuospatial LD* (Cornoldi, Venneri, Marconato, Molin, & Montinari, 2003)—there is one that makes a specific reference to brain functioning: *right-hemisphere developmental LD* (Tranel, Hall, Olson, & Tranel, 1987). In fact, the field of LD has benefited from the rapid advances in behavioral neuroscience that have confirmed the value of applying brain-referenced models to the exploration of behavior in the brain with and without diseases. The application of such models has been partly successful in highlighting the relationship between right-hemisphere mechanisms and the behaviors of individuals who meet NLD criteria. The behaviors associated with right-hemisphere mechanisms include, for example, visuospatial processing, storage and retrieval of visual imagery, aspects of attentional arousal and control, processing of the nonverbal aspects of language (e.g., discourse and prosody), processing of emotionally based stimuli, and processing of tactile stimuli (Lezak, Howieson, & Loring, 2004). The association between right-hemisphere mechanisms and poor nonverbal processing that is seen in the social, behavioral, and organizational disorders has been well documented in direct evidence derived from adult and developmental lesion studies (Brumback & Staton, 1982; Gross-Tsur, Shalev, Manor, & Amir, 1995; Mattson, Sheer, & Fletcher, 1992; Nichelli & Venneri, 1995; Tranel et al., 1987; Voeller, 1986; Weintraub & Mesulam, 1983). In particular, Nichelli and Venneri (1995) reported a case study (AE) of a young man, age 22, with a developmental LD consisting of visuospatial deficits and arithmetic difficulties. In particular, AE made errors in writing multidigit numbers under dictation. In written calculation he gave incorrect answers arising from column confusion. Positron emission tomography (PET) scans revealed a marked hypometabolism of the right hemisphere. Some years later, however, Venneri and other researchers moved the focus on the underlying cognitive processes, and a different label—visuospatial LD—was adopted for referring to children with NLD.

Visuospatial LD

In an attempt to analyze cognitive processes rather than brain functioning, there were researchers who had already focused on the role of visuospatial abilities rather than linguistic deficits. It became evident that visuospatial abilities might be central to explaining differences between children with NLD and other forms of LD. Thus, in considering the relation of LD to visuospatial dysfunction, two subtypes of LD, one associated with weak linguistic abilities and the other with poor visuospatial abilities, emerged (Cornoldi & Soresi, 1980; see also Rourke, 1989).

At the beginning of the 21st century, Cornoldi et al. (2003; see also Mammarella & Cornoldi, 2005a, 2005b) proposed using the term "visuospatial learning disability" (or disorder) rather than NLD for two reasons. First, to establish a crucial criterion for the identification of children with NLD highlighting the role of visuospatial processes as the core deficit; and second, to avoid a vague and unhelpful term for categorizing children with NLD. These researchers argued that most diagnostic labels use terms indicating the presence and not the absence of a difficulty—for example, "specific language impairment" clearly defines the nature of the problem. In contrast, the term "nonverbal learning disability" suggests that there is no problem in the verbal domain, but does not specify the domain of impairment. Nevertheless, the authors abandoned their attempt to redefine the categorical label. The scientific community did not easily associate children with visuospatial LD to NLD and, moreover, it was determined to be too narrow, emphasizing the role of only visuospatial processes while leaving other clinical indices in the shadows.

Different Profiles within NLD

A problem in the field of NLD has been the absence of widely accepted and agreed-upon criteria. Thus, children receiving a diagnosis of NLD seemed to present with differing profiles. A survey study conducted by Solodow et al. (2006) interviewed three groups of experts—educators, clinical psychologists, and neurodevelopmentalists—about the most typical signs characterizing children with NLD. These clinical and educational professionals were then asked to classify different children as having or not having an NLD. The researchers found that the three categories of experts did not completely agree. Specifically, neurodevelopmentalists and clinical therapists were two times more likely to make the diagnosis than were educators. Table 1.2 lists the most

TABLE 1.2. Indicators for NLD Considered by the Groups of Experts Interviewed by Solodow et al. (2006)

- Higher VIQ versus lower PIQ
- Difficulties with visuospatial and visuoperceptual skills
- Weaknesses in visual organization
- Visual memory difficulties
- Difficulty perceiving gestalt
- Poor problem-solving skills
- Problems with nonverbal reasoning
- Inability to determine most salient features
- Poor handwriting or graphomotor difficulties
- Gross motor difficulties
- Difficulty with conceptual math
- Difficulty understanding arithmetic calculations with strong decoding skills

Note. The presentation order represents the importance of the indicator. VIQ, Verbal IQ; PIQ, Performance IQ.

important indicators for diagnosing children with NLD according to these groups of clinicians.

A possible explanation of the absence of complete agreement among different experts may be related to the presence of different profiles within NLD. In particular, some authors (Forrest, 2004; Grodzinsky, Forbes, & Bernstein, 2010) sought different ways to distinguish among different NLD profiles, on the basis of clinical indices—for example, Forrest suggested creating two subtypes. The first would be a visuospatial disability category for children with severe visuospatial deficits affecting their academic achievement, mathematics in particular. The second subtype would be for children whom social skills deficits were most concerning. It was suggested that these categories could be of particular interest for the purposes of treatment. Grodzinsky et al. recommended distinguishing among three subtypes of NLD. A first profile was called *processing speed disorder* and describes children unable to scan and select relevant information efficiently. The second profile, *concept integration disorder,* is similar to Forrest's visuospatial disability. Grodzinsky et al. felt, however, that the term "visuospatial" may create confusion because children with the *concept integration disorder* subtype have difficulty in weaving elements together to create a whole mental representation. They frequently fail in visuoconstructive tests, visuospatial memory tasks, and mathematics. Finally, the third profile was labeled *social adaptation disorder* and refers to children whose social adaptation problems are apparent both at home and at school (see Table 1.3).

Some researchers suggest that children who seem to mainly present with visual and spatial problems can be further differentiated. For example, on the basis of the visuospatial approach, visuospatial working memory (WM) has been considered a critical factor underlying the difficulties encountered by children with NLD, and these children can be differentiated according to the specific aspect of visuospatial WM (VSWM) that is mostly impaired (Cornoldi, dalla Vecchia, & Tressoldi, 1995; Cornoldi, Rigoni, Tressoldi, & Vio, 1999; Cornoldi & Vecchi, 2003). In agreement with the continuity model of WM developed by Cornoldi and Vecchi (2003), WM functions are not rigidly separated. Rather, two fundamental dimensions can be identified: the horizontal continuum, related to the various types of material involved (e.g., verbal, visual, spatial); and the vertical continuum, related

TABLE 1.3. Summary of the Main Different NLD Profiles Described in the Literature

Profiles based on visuospatial working memory	General clinical profiles
Passive versus active: Difficulties in maintaining (passive) or in maintaining and processing (active) visuospatial stimuli	*Visuospatial disability/concept integration disorder*: Severe visuospatial deficits affecting academic achievement and in weaving elements together to create a whole mental representation
Spatial–sequential versus spatial–simultaneous: Difficulties in maintaining the presentation order of spatial locations (spatial–sequential) or in maintaining the configuration of spatial locations simultaneously presented (spatial–simultaneous)	*Social processing disorder/social adaptation disorder*: Difficulties in social adaptation both at home and at school
	Processing speed disorder: Difficulties in selecting relevant information

to the degree of active processing and manipulation of information. Referring to the vertical continuum, Cornoldi, Rigoni, Venneri, and Vecchi (2000) offered evidence based on the observation of single cases, suggesting a dissociation between active and passive VSWM in cases with a diagnosis of NLD. Referring to the horizontal continuum, spatial components have been further distinguished in children with NLD as crucially poor, since a double dissociation has been observed between spatial–sequential WM involved in recalling positions presented one after the other and spatial–simultaneous WM involved in recalling locations simultaneously presented (Mammarella et al., 2006).

Critical Issues Related to the Concept of NLD

The presence of different labels referring to the same disorder—or, by contrast of a unique label referred to different impairments, together with the introduction of multiple profiles—has created a critical concern about the existence of NLD. In the second edition of his book, Pennington (1991) reviewed NLD research and concluded, "In sum, we do not have sufficient evidence to accept it as a valid learning disorder apart from either autism spectrum disorder (ASD), mathematics disorder (MD) or developmental coordination disorder (DCD) all of which are covered in the DSM-IV-TR" (p. 248). A systematic critical review was successively made by Spreen (2011). First, he observed that contrary to expectations, it seems that NLD occurs only quite rarely. Rourke and colleagues would agree on the NLD diagnosis in only 22 cases of their database of 5,000 (i.e., 0.44% of the cases). Yet, Ozols and Rourke (1991) estimate the frequency of NLD in the total LD population as 10%, while Bender and Golden (1990) estimate it at 25%. Spreen (2011) also argues that the inclusion of socioemotional disorders as part of the NLD profile has found only mixed support in the literature. At this time it is questionable whether it can be found in all or even most children with NLD. This would affect the descriptive validity of the NLD diagnosis.

It is worth noting that in the wider practice context, and especially that of the education system, the diagnosis of NLD has gained acceptance in spite of the serious challenges to its validity.

The possible reasons could be summarized as follows. In clinical practice and in educational settings, the group of children who present problems in learning that cannot be related to disturbed language functioning is large. Additionally, until recently, these children needed diagnoses to receive specialized instruction and behavioral interventions in the educational setting. Finally, the number of children in the academic mainstream characterized by behavioral difficulties subsumed under NLD is increasing with resulting attention on educational resources (Grodzinsky et al., 2010).

Wider acceptance of the NLD profile is also documented by the frequency of the diagnostic label and by the presence of popular material and enterprises associated with NLD. At least 14 books for parents and teachers on educating and parenting children with NLD from the year 2000 forward have been published. Moreover, there are different websites for families that provide support and information, indicating that NLD is becoming more commonly diagnosed in school-age children.

Thus, although NLD is not currently recognized by diagnostic manuals, such as *International Classification of Diseases and Related Disorders* (ICD-10; World Health Organization, 1992) and *Diagnostic and Statistical Manual of Mental Disorders* (DSM-5; American Psychiatric Association, 2013), it has nonetheless received a great deal of clinical attention. A goal of many clinicians is to raise awareness of NLD and to eventually have it included in the DSM; however, without a sound body of research to support the diagnosis, this goal may be difficult to achieve. Nonetheless, the increasingly common identification of these children utilizing a "lay diagnosis" (Grodzinsky et al., 2010, p. 434) in the absence of an official DSM diagnosis highlights the need for a review of research literature that could reasonably be applied to school children with learning problems consistent with the popular notion of NLD.

It is worth noting that despite making a specific reference to "learning disability," not all children with a diagnosis of NLD present severe problems with reading, writing, or mathematics severe enough to be considered learning disabled. However, the new diagnostic "specific learning disorder (disability)" in the latest version of the DSM (DSM-5), presents a unique, broader, and more heterogeneous description of children with learning challenges than did previous versions of the DSM. This paradigm shift makes room for the consideration of children who are learning disabled as having an NLD within the category. In any case, research on NLD during the past few years, identified through well-defined criteria, offers a validation of the field. A series of important contributions have moved the field toward a stronger validation of NLD, discussed in subsequent chapters.

CHAPTER TWO

Cognitive and Academic Weaknesses of Children with NLD

In this chapter we review the research on the cognitive weaknesses and learning problems of children with NLD. As we discuss in the fifth chapter, the diagnostic criteria for the identification of children with NLD are mainly focused on the discrepancy between verbal and nonverbal general abilities. Hence, this chapter does not address issues related to general intellectual functioning. Moreover, due to differences in the identification criteria adopted in the reviewed studies, the results illustrated in the present chapter refer to groups that are not fully comparable—a problem that is common to other disorders. For example, Murphy, Mazzocco, Hanich, and Early (2007) showed that the cognitive characteristics of children with mathematics LD varied depending on how the disabilities were defined and with which measures the children's performance was assessed. The same can be said of children with NLD. In the present chapter, studies considering cognitive weaknesses are discussed followed by LD in children with NLD.

Cognitive Characteristics of Children with NLD

Research analyzing cognitive processes in children with NLD is shown in Table 2.1. One can see that some aspects have been less well studied than others. For example, spatial abilities have not been extensively studied because low spatial abilities are considered to be a primary inclusion criterion for identifying children with NLD. In contrast, both verbal and visuospatial short-term and WM have been the focus of several studies. In the following paragraphs, the cognitive challenges of children with NLD that are shown in Table 2.1 are discussed, beginning with more simple functions, such as visual perception, and progressing to complex reasoning.

Visual Perception

Only a few studies considering visual perception performances in children with NLD have been carried out. Despite this scarce evidence, visual perception deficits may be critical in NLD and may partly predict impairment of higher information processing. This hypothesis is coherent with the framework formulated in the Rourke (1995) model speculating that primary neuropsychological deficits lead to secondary deficits, which then lead to tertiary deficits, and so on. According to Rourke, primary neuropsychological deficits include tactile and visual perception, and motor coordination. In turn, secondary deficits include tactile and visual attention, whereas visuospatial memory is considered to be a tertiary deficit.

Rourke (1995) also suggested that children with NLD show impaired discrimination and recognition of visual details and visual relationships. As stated by Rourke, simple visual discrimination, especially for material that can be verbalized such as letters and words, usually approaches normal levels with advancing years, but other perceptual deficits can persist. Despite the fact that there is no evidence that visual acuity is poorer in children with NLD than in typically developing children, it seems that specific sensory processes may be weaker in children with NLD. For example, some unpublished data we have collected seem to suggest that children with NLD are poor at tasks assessing stereopsis, meaning the ability to have fully binocular vision for depth perception and three-dimensional visualization. These results may help explain why children with NLD have particular difficulty in processing three-dimensional stimuli.

Several researchers have shown that a significant perceptual problem in NLD is related to complex visuospatial organizational skills. For example, Chow and Skuy (1999) found that children with NLD were poorer than children with specific language disorder at tasks requiring the recognition of gestalt configurations. Mammarella and Pazzaglia (2010) demonstrated that the difficulties of children with NLD in visual perception were parallel to visual memory deficits, observed using the same stimuli. In addition, Semrud-Clikeman, Walkowiak, Wilkinson, and Christopher (2010a) compared an NLD group with AS and ADHD, and found a specific perceptual difficulty in the NLD group, in this case concerning a spatial feature, as assessed by the Judgment of Line Orientation Test (Benton, Sivan, Hamsher, Varney, & Spreen, 1994). Thus, deficits in perception appear to have been documented via several types of experimental stimuli.

Praxic (Motor Coordination) Abilities

Praxic abilities are defined as motor sequences involved in actions guided by cognitive processes. Clinical and empirical evidence largely supports a relation between motor coordination and visuospatial deficits. It appears within the description of both DCD, which also mentions visuospatial weaknesses especially in adolescence (ICD-10; World Health Organization, 1992), and in the description of NLD, which mentions motor coordination problems (Rourke, 1995; Cornoldi et al., 2003). Therefore, both praxic and spatial abilities are often included in the criteria used for the diagnosis of NLD, and maybe for this reason, motor coordination skills have rarely been a focus of research studies. Yet, researchers have offered contrasting evidence regarding dyspraxia and other motor coordination problems in children with NLD.

Using the Hand Movement subtest of the Kaufman Assessment Battery for Children (K-ABC; Kaufman & Kaufman, 1983), Chow and Skuy (1999) did not find significant differences in the test scores between NLD and specific language disorder groups. Likewise, Semrud-Clikeman, Fine, and Bledsoe (2014), using the Purdue Pegboard Test (Tiffin, 1968), found a weakness of children with NLD compared with controls using only the right hand when they were required to place pegs in holes as quickly as possible. However, in another study using the same test, Semrud-Clikeman et al. (2010b) found weaknesses in children with NLD when coordinating the right and left hands together. Durand (2005) found poor performance in children with NLD at the Purdue Pegboard but no difference with respect to controls in a task that required cutting in between two lines that were in the basic shape of an elephant. In addition, Nichelli and Venneri (1995) described a single case of NLD and found that his performance was poor in a constructional apraxia task. As mentioned in Chapter 1, despite differences in the hypothesized neural correlates, it must be noted that the NLD profile has been compared with Gerstmann syndrome (Gerstmann, 1940) for which digital agnosia is a salient symptom. Gerstmann syndrome is characterized by digital agnosia, dyscalculia, and dysgraphia. Although digital agnosia is often clinically assumed in children with NLD, there are no specific studies that have analyzed this deficit extensively and reliably. Thus, evidence is mixed concerning the motor coordination of children with NLD at this point in time.

Visuoconstructive Abilities

There is evidence that children with NLD are impaired in visuoconstructive abilities. These children have exhibited difficulties in copying as well as retrieving and drawing images from memory (Mammarella et al., 2006; Nichelli & Venneri, 1995; Warren, 2003). Low scores on the Rey Complex Figure Test and the Visual–Motor Integration Test (VMI) have also been observed in children (Mammarella et al., 2006) and in an adult with NLD (Nichelli & Venneri, 1995). Semrud-Clikeman et al. (2010b) compared children with NLD, ADHD, and AS, and found that children with NLD performed lower than the other groups on the VMI and the Rey Complex Figure Test. However, it is important to note that the Rey Complex Figure Test was used as one of many criteria for inclusion in the NLD group in the Semrud-Clikeman study.

Problems with visuoconstruction may be related to praxic tasks, motor coordination, oculomotor integration, perception, and memory of organized visual patterns in children with NLD. The visuoconstructive tasks in which children with NLD encounter particular difficulties require the reconstruction of

fragments belonging to an entire integrated figure. Early literature on NLD often reported a difficulty of these children with
the Object Assembly subtest of the WISC (e.g., Drummond,
Ahmad, & Rourke, 2005), which also involved part-to-whole construction. A similar difficulty in children with NLD compared
with matched neurotypical controls was reported by Cornoldi et
al. (1995) on simple tasks requiring the organization of three to
four puzzle pieces requiring visuospatial WM (VSWM). Notably,
children with high-functioning autism (HFA) are characterized
by a diminished sensitivity to perceptual coherence and a locally
oriented processing to visuospatial material (Caron, Mottron,
Berthiaume, & Dawson, 2006; Happé, 1999); this finding has
been used to hypothesize a partial overlapping between the
two profiles (Ozonoff & Rogers, 2003; Semrud-Clikeman et al.,
2010b). However, the overlap between NLD and HFA has been
partly questioned by recent research (Cardillo, Mammarella,
Basso Garcia, & Cornoldi, 2016).

Spatial Abilities

Spatial weaknesses may represent one of the core weaknesses
of children with NLD, affecting perceptual, comprehension,
memory, and imagery processing of spatial information. Since
spatial weaknesses are used as a main diagnostic criterion for
the identification of NLD, in order to avoid circularity researchers have not systematically examined spatial skills. Thus, a well-
articulated description of the aspects that are mostly impaired
and those that are partly spared is lacking, with a few exceptions.
Given the complexity of the domain of spatial skills, it should be
relevant to examine which aspects are most frequently impaired
in children with NLD. Chow and Skuy (1999) administered the
K-ABC (Kaufman & Kaufman, 1983), showing that children
with NLD were impaired in simultaneous (mainly visuospatial)
and not in successive (mainly verbal) processing tasks. We caution, however, that group comparisons only examine the means
of groups, and individual cases may or may not reveal similar
patterns of weaknesses. In addition, a spatial impairment in
children with NLD is often reported not only with respect to
cognitive laboratory tasks but also with respect to everyday life
situations. For example, orientation difficulties of children with

NLD, especially in unfamiliar environments, are often reported (e.g., Rourke, 1995).

Language and Verbal WM

Children with NLD are typically described as poor in spatial tasks, but good in verbal tasks. However, because language involves a variety of different partially independent aspects, specific language-based difficulties may be found. Examples of difficulty concern prosody, or the tone and cadence of spoken language (Drummond et al., 2005), listening comprehension, and verbal WM. Notably, research concerning verbal WM is partly contradictory. On one hand, Liddell and Rasmussen (2005) observed good performances of children with NLD on the verbal immediate memory index subtests of the Children's Memory Scale (CMS; Cohen, 1997). On the other hand, Chow and Skuy (1999) found impaired performance in one of the two verbal WM tests they designed. In a more recent study, Cornoldi et al. (2003) found that children with NLD were impaired in a digit span but not in a verbal free recall test and a single-case study described by Nichelli and Venneri (1995) also showed poor verbal WM. The reasons for these inconsistencies are yet unclear, as are the processes that may underlie verbal WM deficits in NLD. However, it can be hypothesized that higher-level global processes, such as executive functions that influence general WM capacity, may play a role in various subprocesses of verbal WM, such as are seen in VSWM and short-term memory, discussed below.

Visuospatial WM

According to Logie (1995), VSWM is a specific WM component, responsible for the maintenance and processing of distinct visual (e.g., color, shape, texture) and spatial (e.g., position of an object in space) information. VSWM has been specifically explored in a series of studies concerning children with NLD. Evidence suggests that children with NLD are impaired in both simple storage (i.e., passive short-term memory) and complex-span (i.e., active WM) tasks, but that differing individual specific weaknesses can be found. Simple storage tasks (often defined as short-term memory tasks or passive tasks) refer to the retention of information that must not be modified after encoding, while complex-span tasks (also called "active" or "working memory" tasks) require transformation and manipulation of stored information. We describe in the following sections the results of research in both visuospatial short-term and WM, considered, respectively, passive and active components of VSWM based on the distinction between passive and active tasks proposed by Cornoldi and Vecchi (2003).

Visuospatial Short-Term Memory

Visuospatial short-term memory (VSSTM) tasks can be further articulated in many respects. For example, a main distinction concerns the output requirement: Must the child simply recognize an element from a field, or is he or she required to freely recall and/or reproduce a stimulus? A frequently used test for assessing VSSTM is the Corsi Block-Tapping Task, which requires memory for a sequence of spatial locations via a pointing stimulus and a pointing response (see also Chapter 6). Used for children with NLD, the test is sensitive to weakness in VSSTM (Basso Garcia, Mammarella, Tripodi, & Cornoldi, 2014; Cornoldi et al., 2003; Mammarella & Cornoldi, 2005a, 2005b). The Corsi span is considered a visuospatial analogue of the verbal digit span test because it includes both a forward and backward condition. In the forward condition, the task is to recall a series of positions in the same order as they were presented. In the backward condition, the recall order must be completely reversed from the presented order. Although decreased performance is typically seen in the backward condition for verbal spans (fewer items can be recalled in reverse compared with forward), this decrement is not seen in the spatial Corsi Block-Tapping Task (Farrand & Jones, 1996; Jones, Farrand, Stuart, & Morris, 1995) when a typical population is considered. However, a decreased performance in the backward condition of the Corsi Block-Tapping Task may be a crucial marker of a poor spatial ability (Cornoldi & Mammarella, 2008) and may be found in children with NLD (see Figure 2.1). For example, Mammarella and Cornoldi (2005b), as well as Basso Garcia et al. (2014), compared the forward and backward versions of a digit span test and the Corsi task in children with NLD and in typically developing children. They found

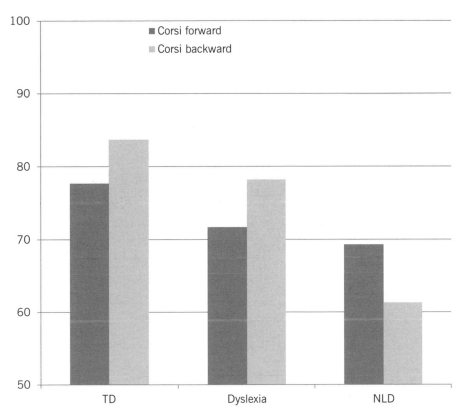

FIGURE 2.1. Proportions of positions correctly remembered in the forward and backward versions of the Corsi Block-Tapping Task by children with typical development (TD), dyslexia, and NLD. Data collected at the Padua, Italy, lab. See also Basso Garcia et al. (2014).

that both groups performed more poorly in the backward version of the digit span, while a forward/backward discrepancy was seen only for the children with NLD in the Corsi Block-Tapping Task. In fact, children with NLD had more difficulty than typically developing children in remembering locations in the backward version. These findings could be interpreted with reference to the hypothesis that the backward Corsi involves spatial–simultaneous processes (see Mammarella & Cornoldi, 2005b; Cornoldi & Mammarella, 2008), by means of which the sequence of blocks is encoded and retained as an overall pattern of locations (i.e., a simultaneous mental representation of the pathway as a whole), thus facilitating its recall starting from the last item.

Given their low visuospatial abilities and poor VSWM, children with NLD may have problems with constructing and retaining a simultaneous representation of a spatial pathway. These results could also be associated with a more general differentiation between spatial–simultaneous processes referring to spatial locations simultaneously presented in a WM task and sequential–spatial encoding in which participants are presented with spatial locations produced sequentially and have to recall previous positions. This recall has been found to be selectively impaired in children with NLD (see Mammarella et al., 2006). However, this association must be cautiously considered because in performing simple VSSTM recognition tasks, children with NLD may be poorer in sequential rather than in simultaneous spatial tasks overall (Mammarella, Lucangeli, & Cornoldi, 2010a). Actually, single cases have been described with deficits associated primarily with either spatial–simultaneous or spatial–sequential processes (Mammarella et al., 2006).

Active VSWM

Increasing evidence is being accumulated that confirms the importance of considering active VSWM for understanding the cognitive impairments of children with NLD (Cornoldi et al., 1995, 1999; Mammarella & Cornoldi, 2005a, 2005b). Active VSWM deficits might explain why children with NLD have difficulty with activities that are assumed to involve information maintained in VSWM such as mathematics, drawing, and spatial orientation. Study of active VSWM in these children might bring a better understanding of the nature of their difficulties and also provide an opportunity to examine the functioning of VSWM.

Concerning the distinction between simple storage (required only to recall information) and complex-span tasks (required both to maintain and process visuospatial information), Cornoldi et al. (2000) described two NLD cases that showed a double dissociation between passive (e.g., simple-span) and active (e.g., complex-span) tasks. Furthermore, within active VSWM, it has been hypothesized that WM difficulties may be associated with failure to control irrelevant information. This hypothesis was applied to the case of children with NLD's active VSWM by Mammarella and Cornoldi (2005a). They presented a selective VSWM task to three groups: children with NLD, children with specific language weaknesses, and typically developing children. In the task, matrices of progressively increasing length that included one or more colored cells were shown. For each matrix, sequences of locations were presented and participants had to recall only the last location of each sequence. As a secondary task, participants had to press a key when a location corresponded to a colored cell (see Figure 2.2). It was found that children with NLD were poor at the task compared with the other groups. An important finding of this research was that the weaker performance of the NLD group at the VSWM task was associated with specific patterns of errors, in particular the erroneous recall of irrelevant information, thus involving a malfunctioning of highest-level attentional control. Children with NLD not only gave a lower number

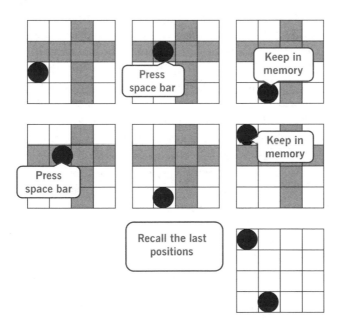

FIGURE 2.2. An example of material proposed in a selective VSWM task. The recall of the last-presented positions is considered to be a correct response, the recall of previously presented positions is considered to be an intrusion error, and the recall of nonpresented positions is considered to be an invention error.

of correct responses than the other groups, but also responded with a greater number of intrusions (gave more frequently as an incorrect response an already presented position, for example, they recalled the first cell in the third row, in the set presented in Figure 2.2) than invention errors (incorrect never-presented positions). In contrast, the other two groups made an equal number of intrusion and invention errors. A further aspect relating to VSWM (Cornoldi & Vecchi, 2003) is mental imagery; due to its importance and partial autonomy, we treat it in a separate section below.

Mental Imagery

Within cognitive psychology, imagery has been investigated mainly in two different ways. The first examines mental imagery as a dependent, subjective, measurable variable. It studies qualitative subjective aspects of imagery and the extent to which mental images are subjectively similar to the physical objects that are being imagined. The second concerns the use of mental images as independent variables (manipulated by researchers) in which observable aspects are reflected in behaviors and especially in the performance of participants (Richardson, 1999). These two aspects of mental imagery may not coincide, as it has been observed that sometimes individuals poor in objective mental imagery tasks may nonetheless report vivid mental images and vice versa.

We focus here only on the few studies that collect objective measures of mental imagery. Given the presumed relation between VSWM and visuospatial mental imagery it is not surprising that children with NLD are also poor at mental imagery tasks. For example, Cornoldi et al. (1999) and Cornoldi and Guglielmo (2001) systematically studied the mental imagery abilities of children with NLD and found a general impairment of imagery performance. Tasks requiring either the scanning of mental images, or the creation of interactive images, were difficult for children with NLD.

In another study, Cornoldi, Ficili, Giofrè, Mammarella, and Mirandola (2011) proposed a mental pathway task (see Figure 2.3) to three groups of adolescents ages 13–17: an NLD group, a group with depressive symptoms, and a control group. Participants were invited to imagine either a bidimensional or a

3 × 3 × 3 Matrix   5 × 5 Matrix

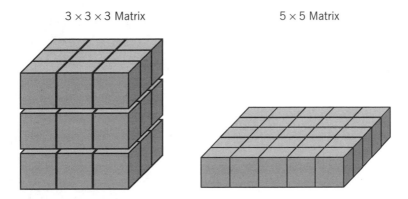

FIGURE 2.3. Example of matrices used in the mental pathway task.

three-dimensional matrix with a series of cells (e.g., a simple 5 × 5 board or a 3 × 3 × 3 three-dimensional matrix). The children then had to imagine following a pathway on the matrix in correspondence with verbal instructions (e.g., "Go left, down") and point, on request, to the position reached at the end of the instructions on a corresponding blank matrix. The researchers found that this task successfully discriminated the strengths and deficits of mental imagery in children with NLD. These children demonstrated particular difficulty with the three-dimensional matrix (Cornoldi et al., 2011).

Executive Functions

A review of the literature on NLD found that most researchers included measures of visuomotor integration, social functioning, and mathematics, while few included direct measures of executive functioning (Fine et al., 2013). Nonetheless, executive functions should be hypothesized as a set of processes involved in the NLD profile (e.g., as proposed in Meltzer's [2007] book). In particular, it is unknown whether—due to their specific visuospatial weakness—children with NLD experience difficulty with executive tasks specifically requiring the processing of visuospatial information, or conversely whether such deficits are global and not affected by the nature of the presented material.

With the exception of the particular executive function represented by active VSWM, literature assessing executive functions in NLD is too scarce to definitively distinguish between modal and global deficits. In an old study, Fisher, Deluca, and Rourke (1997) observed that children with NLD performed poorly compared with children with a verbal LD on the Wisconsin Card Sorting Test. In another study, Semrud-Clikeman and coauthors (2014) collected three measures of executive functioning using the Delis–Kaplan Tests of Executive Functioning (D-KEFS; Delis, Kaplan, & Kramer, 2001) and observed differences among children with NLD, children with AS, and controls, especially at the trail-making task, an activity that appears to involve VSWM and sequencing.

Long-Term Memory

Evidence regarding long-term memory (LTM) functioning in children with NLD is scarce and unclear. Only one study (Fisher & Deluca, 1997) reported impairment in NLD related to organization of verbal material for retrieval, based on the administration of the California Verbal Learning Test (CVLT-C; Delis, Kramer, Kaplan, & Ober, 1994). In this task, examinees are rewarded for using a categorization strategy to recall lists of words. However, an alternative explanation to poor LTM may be that mental representation of objects to support LTM (e.g., fruits, toys) might be the critical component influencing LTM in the NLD population. In another study, Liddell and Rasmussen (2005) used the CMS (Cohen, 1997) subtests for short- and long-term verbal and visuospatial memory tasks. They found that children with NLD had difficulty with both short- and long-term visuospatial tasks, whereas verbal LTM was commensurate with typically developing children.

Reasoning

Difficulty in visuospatial reasoning in the presence of good verbal performance is implicit in the main criteria adopted for the diagnosis of NLD; therefore, reasoning has not been systematically studied in NLD. Chow and Skuy (1999) found an NLD impairment in visuospatial but not in verbal reasoning tasks; their results have been supported by a few subsequent studies. One study found a specific difficulty in the NLD group compared

TABLE 2.1. Cognitive Abilities Analyzed in Different Research Studies Examining the Performance of Children with NLD

Cognitive processes	1	2	3	4	5	6	7	8	9	10	11	12	13	14	15	16	17	18
Visual perception		−											−		−		−	
Praxic abilities		+					−								−			+/−
Visuoconstructive abilities														−	−		−	
Spatial abilities		−																
Verbal working memory		+/−			+/−					+					+			
Visuospatial short-term memory	−			−	−					−		−	−		−			
Visuospatial working memory				−							−			−				
Mental imagery			−	−		−												
Executive functions									−						−			+/−
Long-term memory								−		+/−					+			
Reasoning		−														+/−	−	+/−

Note. Numbers in the column heads refer to the following studies: (1) Basso Garcia et al. (2014); (2) Chow and Szuy (1999); (3) Cornoldi and Guglielmo (2001); (4) Cornoldi et al. (1999); (5) Cornoldi et al. (2003); (6) Cornoldi et al. (2011); (7) Durand (2005); (8) Fisher and DeLuca (1997a); (9) Fisher, DeLuca, and Rourke (1997); (10) Liddell and Rasmussen (2005); (11) Mammarella and Cornoldi (2005a); (12) Mammarella and Cornoldi (2005b); (13) Mammarella and Pazzaglia (2010); (14) Mammarella et al. (2006); (15) Nichelli and Venneri (1995); (16) Schiff et al. (2009); (17) Semrud-Clikeman et al. (2010a); (18) Semrud-Clikeman et al. (2014). −, presence of a deficit; +/−, no clear evidence of a deficit; +, presence of a strength.

with children with verbal LD at a task involving visuospatial reasoning and fine-motor coordination skills (Schiff, Bauminger, & Toledo, 2009). In contrast, the two groups performed similarly to each other in a task involving the abstract representation of two stories. Fluid reasoning subtests and a test of spatial reasoning were administered by Semrud-Clikeman et al. (2010a) using the Woodcock–Johnson Cognitive III (WJ-Cog III; Woodcock, McGrew, & Mather, 2001), and a weaker performance both in children with NLD and children with AS was observed compared with children with ADHD or typically developing children. However, 4 years later Semrud-Clikeman and colleagues (2014) administered the same tasks to another sample and observed that the NLD group performed more poorly than did other groups only at the spatial relations task, thus finding further support of the hypothesis that NLD weaknesses in reasoning tasks are mainly related to the manipulation of visuospatial information.

Academic Performance of Children with NLD

As mentioned in Chapter 1 and as the name of the disorder suggests, the study of NLD originated from the analysis of specific academic difficulties presented by children who showed cognitive weaknesses in the nonverbal domains rather than in verbal domains. In fact, Johnson and Myklebust (1967) included the subgroup of NLD in their influential presentation of LD, and Rourke and Finlayson (1975) found a specific nonverbal weakness in a subgroup of children with calculation difficulties compared with children with reading decoding difficulties. Subsequently, the focus on these children's characteristics progressively shifted to the associated cognitive processes, reducing attention to school learning aspects. However, the discrepancy between reading decoding (good) and calculation (poor) has been used in most of the research as a criterion for diagnosing children with NLD and this may create confusion as it is obvious in these studies that children with NLD present specific patterns of performance in reading and calculation as per the group definition. For this reason, we next pay particular attention to aspects of the academic performance of children with NLD that were not part of the diagnostic process.

Reading Decoding and Spelling

As previously mentioned, reading decoding (i.e., how fluently and accurately verbal material is read) is typically good in children with NLD, although Rourke (1995) reports that, due to the visual aspects associated with the acquisition of letter form–sound relationship, NLD may present difficulties in the early phases of reading decoding. Reading decoding has also been examined in studies by Gross-Tsur et al. (1995) and Semrud-Clikeman et al. (2010a), which further confirmed good performances of children with NLD. Moreover, additional studies (Cornoldi et al., 2000; Mammarella et al., 2006) have offered descriptions of cases with NLD, which included measures of spelling that resulted in typically good skill development (see Table 2.2).

Language Comprehension

Although most researchers have focused on examination and demonstration of visuospatial deficits of children with NLD, these children also seem to exhibit particular linguistic deficits. Indeed, the language of such individuals may be moderately to severely deficient in content and pragmatics. Pragmatics refers to the functional and contextual aspects of language, including an appreciation of the rules of social discourse, the speaker's purpose for communication, and how language is modified to fit different situations (Boone & Plante, 1993). Children with NLD may be deficient in this dimension of language; many of them demonstrate characteristics of verbosity, poor prosody, and low appreciation of the social discourse rules (Rourke & Tsatsanis, 1996).

Support for Rourke's (1995) hypothesis that language comprehension may be impaired was offered by Humphries, Cardy, Worling, and Peets (2004), who showed the presence of both narrative comprehension and retelling difficulties in a sample of children with NLD. The narrative performance of the NLD group was not significantly different from that of children with verbal impairment on all the comprehension or story-retelling measures collected in this study, but children with NLD performed more poorly than typically developing children in comprehending inferences. Other studies seem to suggest that language comprehension difficulties in children with NLD are related in particular to the processing of spatial information.

Worling, Humphries, and Tannock (1999) found that children with NLD have difficulty with language inferencing, specifically when dependent on appreciation of spatial relationships, suggesting that children with NLD have difficulty in developing spatial representations or spatial mental models (Johnson-Laird, 1983).

Some studies examined comprehension, memory, drawings, and object locations based on descriptions of spatial relationships and found that children with NLD may have difficulty in understanding spatial descriptions. In one study, children with NLD were presented with spatial descriptions and they had to relocate the landmarks in a background (Rigoni, Cornoldi, & Alcetti, 1997). The image in Figure 2.4 shows the representation made by a child who was not able to relocate the landmarks: in fact, the text described a square with a fountain in the center, an arch at a corner, and a car and a dog between the arch and the fountain. The child failed to correctly represent all the spatial relationships and even located the car in an impossible position, demonstrating his low ability to understand and represent spatial relationships. In a further study, Mammarella et al. (2009b) used spatial descriptions, one regarding survey (i.e., providing an overview of the spatial layout, using terms such as "north," "south," and so on), and one regarding route (i.e., considering

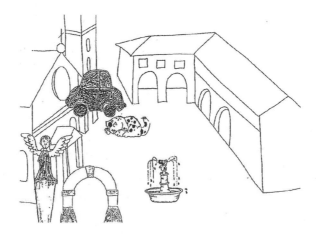

FIGURE 2.4. Example of a spatial representation made by a child with NLD. The child must locate the pictures of the objects on a sheet containing the drawing of the square on the basis of the following description: "In the square there is a fountain in the center, a statue in a corner, and an arch close to the statue, and between the arch and the fountain there are a car and a dog."

the point of view of a person moving within the environment) perspective, and observed poor performances of children with NLD in survey descriptions. In a successive study, Mammarella, Meneghetti, Pazzaglia, and Cornoldi (2015) replicated this observation, but also found that children with NLD, when compared with children with a reading disability, did not take advantage of the availability of the text during a comprehension task as well. In conclusion, these findings support the hypothesis that children with NLD show difficulties in the ability to process and graphically represent spatial descriptions. This difficulty is particularly evident when children with NLD must process survey descriptions (see Table 2.2).

Handwriting

Handwriting difficulties have not been extensively studied in children with NLD. Clinical evidence seems to suggest that children with NLD may encounter problems with handwriting, specifically graphomotor skills. This is also consistent with the observation of a frequent fine-motor coordination problem in children with NLD. However, only Gross-Tsur et al. (1995) tested handwriting in children with NLD, reporting that six out of 20 of these children had graphomotor problems.

Calculation

Poor mathematics competence is often considered a critical index of NLD, but the various mathematics skills—such as number sense, arithmetic fact retrieval, mental and written calculation, and so on—have largely gone unspecified; mathematics skills have been globally considered. For example, in their first studies, Rourke and Finlayson (1978) focused on two groups of children with mathematics impairments: children with poor mathematics skills but with reading skills appropriate for their chronological age, and children performing poorly in both mathematics and reading tasks. They found that only the first group presented a specific visuospatial (nonverbal) problem. A relation between visuospatial problems and weaknesses in number processing, or more specifically with the discrimination of numerosity, has also been found in children with a diagnosis of developmental dyscalculia (Iuculano, Tang, Hall, & Butterworth,

2008; Landerl, Fussenegger, Moll, & Willburger, 2009). In addition, the link between visuospatial functioning and mathematics has also been confirmed by the presence of spatial acalculia in adult patients with brain lesions who have difficulties with considering the relative positions and order of digits (Hécaen, Angelergues, & Houiller, 1961).

Thus, although it is generally recognized that children with NLD perform well in reading and poorly in mathematics (Forrest, 2004), calculation skills have only occasionally been studied in depth. It must be noted that mathematics difficulties seen in this population may be related to VSWM impairments rather than to number sense. Venneri, Cornoldi, and Garuti (2003) compared children with NLD and controls in arithmetic calculations, finding the most severe NLD group's difficulties in written calculation. The authors hypothesized that children with NLD do not have a generalized difficulty with calculation per se; their problems should emerge instead when dealing with specific spatial processes, including VSWM, which support calculation. This hypothesis was confirmed by Mammarella et al. (2010a) in children with symptoms of NLD, whose performance was impaired at written calculation (see examples of errors in Figure 2.5) and number-ordering tasks. Covariance analyses showed that these VSWM impairments were more important than the children's calculation weaknesses. Finally, Bachot, Gevers, Fias, and Royers (2005) found no signs of the typical spatial–numerical association of response codes (SNARC) effect (i.e., the preference for

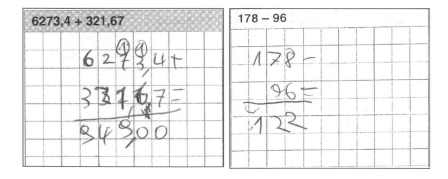

FIGURE 2.5. Examples of written calculation errors found in children with NLD.

left-hand responses to small numbers and right-hand responses to large numbers; see Hubbard, Piazza, Pinel, & Dehaene, 2005, for a review) when children with NLD were compared with typically developing children. As the SNARC effect is associated with the hypothesis that the sequence of numbers is spatially represented along a mental number line, the authors concluded that poor visuospatial competence may produce a basic abnormality in representing numerical magnitudes on a mental number line, suggesting that this may contribute to NLD numerical disabilities. Arithmetic competencies of children with NLD were also studied by Mammarella et al. (2013a), who found that these children were impaired at a task requiring comparison of the numerosity of dots, while children with comorbid dyscalculia and dyslexia showed low performances in arithmetic facts retrieval, which is supported by verbal WM processes (see Table 2.2).

To summarize, calculation difficulties of children with NLD have been found in the following areas:

- Written calculation (in particular with carry/borrow procedure)
- Column alignment
- SNARC effect
- Dots comparison
- Number ordering

Geometry

Geometry skills in children with NLD have been investigated in only one research study to date (Mammarella, Giofrè, Ferrara, & Cornoldi, 2013b), although it is plausible that, given their low visuoconstructive skills and visuospatial abilities, this might be an area of particular difficulty. However, an important point to be considered when examining the relationship between geometry and underlying cognitive processes is that geometry is a broad area with many facets not exclusively visuospatial. In fact, geometric competence can involve both intuitive concepts (intuitive geometry), as well as aspects more associated with schooling. The concept of *intuitive geometry* has been recently introduced by Dehaene, Izard, Pica, and Spelke (2006); they investigated whether some principles of geometry can be considered as core

TABLE 2.2. Learning Difficulties Analyzed in Different Research Studies Examining Performance of Children with NLD

Learning difficulties	1	2	3	4	5	6	7	8	9	10	11	12	13
Reading decoding			+								+		
Language comprehension				–		–			–	–			–
Handwriting			–										
Arithmetic/calculation	–	–	–		–		–				–	–	
Geometry								–					

Note. Numbers in the column heads refer to the following studies. (1) Bachot et al. (2005); (2) Forrest (2004); (3) Gross-Tsur et al. (1995); (4) Humphries et al. (2004); (5) Mammarella et al. (2013a); (6) Mammarella et al. (2009b); (7) Mammarella et al. (2010a); (8) Mammarella et al. (2013b); (9) Mammarella et al. (2015); (10) Semrud-Clikeman and Glass (2008); (11) Semrud-Clikeman et al. (2010a); (12) Venneri et al. (2003); (13) Worling et al. (1999). –, presence of a deficit; +, presence of a strength.

culture-free concepts (see also Spelke, Lee, & Izard, 2010) by examining the spontaneous geometric knowledge of an Amazonian native group that was not exposed to geometric instruction. They found that the Amazonian native group succeeded remarkably well with intuitive concepts of geometry and so the researchers consequently considered these concepts as primitive core concepts of geometry. Mammarella et al. (2013b) used the same material as Dehaene and colleagues and tested a group of children with NLD and found that this group performed more poorly than controls. Although this result may seem rather obvious, as geometry has an evident visuospatial component and children with NLD are characterized by a visuospatial weakness, it had never been documented. In addition, the authors observed that a VSWM deficit explained the difficulty of children with NLD, but not of typically developing controls, in intuitive geometry, suggesting that for the NLD group the involvement of VSWM in the acquisition of basic intuitive concepts is crucial. In fact, when the differences were controlled for VSWM tasks using VSWM as the covariate, the difference in intuitive geometry between groups disappeared, confirming that a spatial WM difficulty may be primary in children with NLD and also mediates their difficulties in intuitive geometry.

Conclusions

This chapter reviewed selected studies that examined the underlying cognitive/neuropsychological processes and academic performances of children with NLD. As we have seen, research was mainly oriented in studying the cognitive and academic challenges of this group of children and, for this reason, one may have the impression that children with NLD present only weaknesses. However, the NLD profile also presents strengths that may produce important outcomes in real-life situations, as we have seen from the examples of famous writers (see Chapter 1), which may be used for developing strategies to compensate for their weaknesses. This point is treated more in depth in Chapter 7 in which intervention strategies are discussed.

CHAPTER THREE

Emotional and Social Difficulties of Children with NLD

During recent decades the importance of emotional and social functioning to academic success and life adjustment has gained traction (Linnenbrink, 2006). Researchers have found that psychosocial factors such as belonging (Bond et al., 2007; Walton & Cohen, 2011), self-concept (Marsh & Martin, 2011), and social skill (Raver et al., 2011) can influence school performance as well as physical and mental health outcomes. Vulnerable students, such as those with minority or immigrant status (Walton & Cohen, 2007) and learning challenges (McDougall, DeWitt, King, Miller, & Killip, 2007), appear to be at greatest risk for social maladjustment. However, they seem to gain from interventions that target the social and emotional factors related to school and peer relations (Walton & Cohen, 2011).

The neural and behavioral processes involved in emotional and social functioning are still being discovered, but several cognitive-behavioral models have been proposed. Among the most utilized is Crick and Dodge's (1994) model of social processing, which outlines the cognitive steps and the behavioral actions involved in first recognizing social stimuli all the way through finally performing an appropriate response. In this model, social processing begins when a child recognizes a social cue at the sensory level. Before an action is performed, the cue must be interpreted based on prior knowledge, current intent or goals, and biases related to how the intents of others are perceived (see

Figure 3.1). Although there are many additional steps and inter-related processes in this model, most of the social functioning research in NLD has assumed that a breakdown is evident at the initial encoding stages—for example, in recognizing facial expressions and kinesthetic "body language" cues. Additional research has focused on the self-regulatory and attentional aspects of social functioning, and most recently, memory has been implicated. Finally, there has been historical concern regarding the psychological and emotional adjustment of persons with NLD. The following sections provide a brief overview of the historical research on social and emotional symptoms in NLD followed by

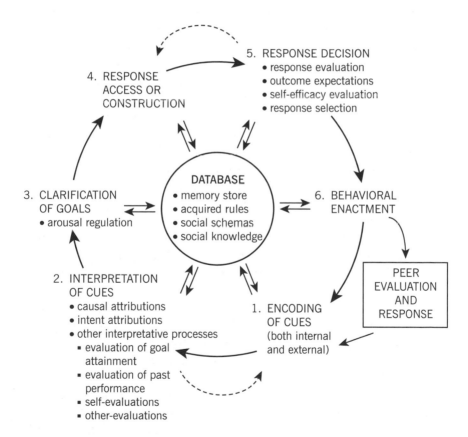

FIGURE 3.1. A reformulated social information-processing model of children's social adjustment. From Crick and Dodge (1994). Copyright 1994 by the American Psychological Association. Reprinted by permission.

a discussion of specific findings related to social cue encoding and interpretation, attention, memory, and psychological adjustment in persons with NLD.

A Brief Historical Perspective

As early as the 1960s, Johnson and Myklebust (1967) theorized that children with nonverbal learning deficits could have difficulty with social perception as well as regulation of attention and self-monitoring. They defined social perception as the ability to adapt and to anticipate the consequences of one's own behavior in response to socially relevant information, and they suggested that there is a secondary deficit in this domain for children with NLD. Subsequently, Rourke expanded this idea in his influential delineation of the NLD profile (e.g., Rourke, 1989).

Rourke's initial conceptualization of NLD did not include social problems as a primary characteristic. Rather he supposed that social and emotional difficulties were downstream effects of various constellations of primary, secondary, and tertiary assets, and deficits associated with NLD (Rourke, 1995). Specifically, problems in social competence, emotional stability, and adaptation to novel stimuli were identified as deficit areas arising from problems in visual and tactile perception, attention, and memory, which in combination could result in poor interpretation of social information (Fine & Semrud-Clikeman, 2010; Rourke, 1989). This perspective delineated a theoretical boundary between autism and NLD because social symptoms in ASD were assumed to be a primary required feature of the autism phenotype. Nonetheless, many researchers have noted the similarity between NLD and HFA (also known as Asperger syndrome [AS]) particularly in regard to difficulties with nonverbal communication and the ability to maintain friendships (Rourke, 2000).

One of the issues confounding research on social functioning in NLD is this symptomatic proximity to the autism spectrum. Early research comprised case studies, small samples, and diagnostic criteria that most likely captured many children with autism who also displayed verbal strength, such as those with AS (according to earlier versions of the DSM; see Fine et al., 2013, for a critical review). In a recent study involving more than 100 children, more than 30% of the children previously diagnosed with NLD who self-referred to a research study on NLD met criteria for AS or HFA based on DSM-IV-TR and Autism Diagnostic Interview—Revised criteria (Jodene Goldenring Fine, personal data). Thus, the social functioning symptoms of NLD may be significantly heterogeneous depending on whether a diagnosis of ASD could better describe a portion of the research population.

Despite these challenges, recent research—in combination with the historical work largely performed by Rourke and his colleagues—provides some information on the social and emotional functioning of children with NLD. In his books, Rourke (1989, 1995) highlighted the presence of socioemotional and adaptation deficits of children with NLD. Specifically, he listed clinical observations concerning weaknesses in the following social aspects:

- Adaptation in novel situation: defined as a difficulty in organizing, analyzing, and synthesizing novel complex situations with a presence of rote and inappropriate behaviors.
- Social competence: defined as a difficulty in social perceptions, social judgments, and social interactions with a tendency of social isolation with advancing years.
- Emotional disturbance: defined as a high risk in developing internalized forms of psychopathology, such as anxiety and depression (see also Casey et al., 1991; Fuerst, & Rourke, 1993).
- Activity level: defined as a presence of hyperactive behaviors during early childhood and hypoactivity with advancing years.

According to Rourke's (1989) conceptualization, children with NLD fail to understand nonverbal communicative messages, such as facial expressions and body language, and also have difficulty in estimating the space between themselves and other people, both physically and psychologically. As a result, these children may attempt to throw themselves into a situation without considering the consequences of their behavior. He observed that, much like children with autism, children with NLD feel more comfortable in speaking and interacting with adults or with younger children than with same-age peers.

With regard to psychological adjustment, Rourke hypothesized that individuals with profiles associated with NLD present serious risks of psychological disorders. For example, using the Personality Inventory for Children (PIC; Wirt, Lachar, Klinedinst, & Seat, 1977) as the measure of psychiatric symptoms, Fuerst, Fisk, and Rourke (1990) found that children with poorer nonverbal than verbal skills were more likely to show severe psychopathology compared with children with equivalent or greater Performance IQ (PIQ) than Verbal IQ (VIQ) WISC (Wechsler, 1949) scores. Specifically, there were a significantly greater number of children with VIQ > PIQ by at least 10 WISC standard scale points appearing in the externalizing group ($p < .05$), but no significantly greater number assigned to the internalizing group ($p = .13$) based on raw count classification. Analyses to examine the relation between degree of VIQ–PIQ discrepancy and pathology were not conducted. Subsequently, in a review analyzing the social–emotional and behavioral domains, Little (1993) concluded that "there is some support for the hypothesis that individuals with NLD may be at greater risk than other children with LD for both internalized and externalized forms of psychopathology and social problems" (p. 662), although little strong empirical support for this statement was evident at that time.

Successively, Rourke and colleagues (Tsatsanis, Fuerst, & Rourke, 1997) found some weak evidence for internalizing psychopathology in NLD in the same, but expanded, clinical group (Jodene Goldenring Fine, personal communication with Byron Rourke, August 2010) described in the study above. Children with WISC VIQ > PIQ discrepancies were evaluated on the PIC. A 10-point discrepancy was used to describe three basic subgroups, which included VIQ > PIQ, VIQ = PIQ, and VIQ < PIQ, as well as performance below the 30th percentile on at least one subtest of the Wide Range Achievement Test (WRAT; Jastak & Jastak, 1965). All of the children had a WISC Full Scale IQ of at least 80 and were presumed to be learning disabled. The distribution of IQ discrepancy subtypes across mild, moderate, and severe degrees of psychopathology based on the PIC were observed. Although all of the children in the sample were clinically referred—thus there is the expectation that they had learning and/or behavioral difficulties severe enough to warrant assessment—nearly one-half of them were found to have no or only mild psychosocial concerns. Furthermore, no significant differences in psychopathology were found between groups based on WRAT reading, arithmetic, and spelling scores. However, when formulating groups based on the discrepancy between reading and arithmetic or spelling and arithmetic scores, more children with severe psychopathology had the largest gap between verbal and mathematics skills. This finding was not statistically significant and may be overemphasized without warrant. Nonetheless, Tsatsanis et al. (1997) concluded that "children with LD who evidence relatively well-developed rote verbal skills were more likely to demonstrate severe psychopathology" (p. 500). The authors indicated that a particular type of psychosocial functioning (the Internalized Psychopathology subtype) was found to be associated with higher VIQ as compared with PIQ on the WISC.

Historically, there is one case study that has influenced subsequent popular assumptions regarding the psychological adjustment of persons with NLD. In 1989, Rourke, Young, and Leenaars published a case study of a young woman with NLD who had a history of attempted suicide. This study generated discussion over a possible predisposition in NLD for suicide that has reverberated through the decades, alarming parents and teachers alike. Despite the speculative nature of the journal article, and a lack of consideration of other important factors (e.g., comorbid psychiatric conditions, familial patterns, risk/resilience variables), the authors concluded that adults with NLD, "are particularly at risk" (p. 173) compared with other learning-disabled persons. A subsequent literature review, conducted as early as 1993, called into question the dire predictions regarding NLD psychopathology. In her review of the early literature, Little (1993) noted conflicting findings, poor study design, and in particular a lack of control groups, noting that (1) other researchers had found similar life challenges and psychosocial stressors attributed to NLD in Rourke's case study in persons with verbal learning challenges, and (2) research data suggest "no correlation between pattern of verbal versus performance abilities and depression" (p. 659).

Despite the limitations of the historical research discussed above, the contribution of early researchers to our understanding of NLD is to be admired and recognized as the foundation upon which modern research rests. During the past decade, newer research into the emotional and/or psychosocial functioning of children with NLD has emerged (e.g., Mirandola, Losito,

Ghetti, & Cornoldi, 2014). The use of control groups, larger sample sizes, and more rigorous statistical methods have improved the reliability of the findings. Yet there are few studies and some confounding results regarding whether children with NLD are more likely to experience psychological disorders or social deficits more severely than are children with other types of LD. With regard to social functioning, most researchers looked for specific differences at the encoding and interpretation stages of social information processing.

Social Cue Encoding and Interpretation

The Crick and Dodge (1994) social processing model suggests that encoding and interpreting social cues involve many processes including situational analysis (e.g., considering the context in which the cue takes place), assessing the attributions of self and others, and predicting what might happen next, all of which require access to a LTM store of prior knowledge. From a research angle, the encoding and interpretation processes have been primarily assessed by asking persons to verbally interpret the emotions of others from photographs of faces, voice prosody (tone and cadence), and/or situational video vignettes. Not all of these methods are equivalent. For example, interpreting a happy or sad face can be accomplished using a cognitive matching technique (e.g., "upturned mouth = happy," or "furrowed brow = angry"). Interpreting social cues that are embedded in real-time video is thought to be a more difficult, naturalistic task (Fine, Semrud-Clikeman, & Zhu, 2009). Studies from the past two decades have used these techniques to examine social–emotional cue interpretation in children with NLD (see Table 3.1).

Three studies testing the ability to interpret and recognize facial expressions in children with NLD have been published: Dimitrovsky, Spector, Levy-Shiff, and Vakil (1998) and Bloom and Heath (2010) used Pictures of Facial Affect (PFA; Ekman & Friesen, 1976) to measure the interpretation of facial expressions. The PFA is a series of 110 black-and-white photographs of Caucasian adults who were asked to display seven expressions: anger, disgust, fear, happiness, sadness, surprise, and a neutral state.

The Dimitrovsky et al. (1998) study is worth describing in detail because it has been much cited as evidence that children with NLD perceive and interpret faces more poorly than do children with verbal or global learning deficits. However, the conclusions of the authors may have been overstated due to methodological issues. The study used an abbreviated version of the PFA consisting of 48 slides (no neutral faces). All noncontrol children in the study were previously characterized as learning disabled by their schools and demonstrated academic performance 2 years behind their peers, but the specific subjects were not revealed. Children with NLD were identified using a discrepancy between scores on the Rey Auditory Verbal Learning Test, which is a list-learning memory test, and the Benton Visual Retention Test, a test of visual discrimination and short-term (15-second) memory for abstract geometric designs. Classification of children was based on simple cutoffs, with "verbal disabled" (VD) having less than 0 standard z-scores (mean = 0, standard deviation = 1) on the verbal memory test and scores greater than 0 on the visual test, while the "nonverbal-disabled" (NVD) group demonstrated scores less than 0 on the visual and greater than 0 on the verbal test. A group with both scores below 0 was labeled as "both deficits" (BD). Notably, this method can produce an NVD or VD group member with a less than 0.2 standard deviation difference between verbal and visual scores.

No information was given regarding the amount of discrepancy observed for each group. A control nondisabled group was included. No group differences were found for the happy and sad conditions but nondisabled children were significantly better than all learning-disabled groups in identifying surprise. Anger, fear, and disgust were more complex—nondisabled children were better than the NVD and BD groups in identifying anger and fear, but there were no other significant differences (VD was not different from either the NVD/BD or nondisabled groups). For disgust, the NVD group was significantly worse than both the nondisabled and VD groups. To summarize, the NVD group was significantly worse than the VD group only in the disgust condition. Notably, there was also an age effect for the disgust condition, with younger children finding this emotion to be more difficult; there were more than twice as many young children in the NVD group than the VD group. Age was not controlled for in the analysis. Thus, the strongest finding of this paper is that all children with LD perform more poorly in adult facial emotion recognition than do their nondisabled peers (see also Fine et al., 2013).

Working with adolescents, Bloom and Heath (2010) examined facial affect recognition also using a 48-slide abbreviated PFA adult face pool of stimuli. Similar to the Dimitrovsky et al. (1998) study, the neutral condition was not included. In this study, classification into groups was based on average IQ and a one standard deviation discrepancy between reading and arithmetic skills. Results indicated that those with general LD—in other words those with average IQ but poor academics in both reading *and* mathematics—less accurately recognized and interpreted facial expressions compared with those with NLD and typically developing adolescents. There were no statistical differences between the performances of the NLD and typically developing groups. The authors suggest that it may be the severity, rather than the type, of learning challenge that most influences the ability to interpret facial affect (Bloom & Heath, 2010). There is evidence from studies on ADHD that a developmental lag rather than specific neural differences may account for some symptoms in neurodevelopmental disorders (Shaw et al., 2011). A social developmental lag might contribute to delayed neural subprocesses that are needed for facial recognition at a general level. As a matter of conjecture, Bloom and Heath suggest that delays in metacognition may contribute to poor facial recognition.

Another research method was used by Petti, Voelker, Shore, and Hayman-Abello (2003), with somewhat stronger results specific to NLD. The Diagnostic Analysis of Nonverbal Accuracy (DANVA; Nowicki & Duke, 1994) evaluates four basic emotions (happy, sad, anger, fear) using three conditions: faces, gestures (body, no faces), and auditory only. In the auditory-only condition, neutral sentences are read ("I am going out of the room now and I will be back later") using a tone of voice consistent with each of the four emotions. The auditory "paralanguage" condition uses adult voices, while the photographic conditions have one-half child and one-half adult models. Using these stimuli, Petti and colleagues evaluated 11 children with NLD, 11 with verbal LD, and 11 psychiatric but non-LD controls. All of the children were drawn from psychiatric facilities. The researchers matched groups for gender and there were no significant differences in age among groups. All children had Full Scale IQ scores above 80, but children with NLD were required to have VIQ greater than PIQ by at least 12 points, as well as WRAT-R (Jastak, 1984). arithmetic scores at least one standard deviation less than their VIQ score. Results demonstrated that the NLD group was less accurate than the other groups in identifying emotions from body gestures and from adult, but not child, facial emotions and there were no group differences in the interpretation of voices. Thus, this work suggests that children with NLD might have some weakness in the encoding or interpretation of visual, but not verbal, emotional information.

In a study using naturalistic video vignettes of children interacting with one another (Semrud-Clikeman et al., 2014)—the Child and Adolescent Social Perception (CASP) measure (Magill-Evans, Koning, Cameron-Sadava, & Manyk, 1995, 1996)—children with NLD were found to have a similar ability in recognizing emotions in the actors as their typically developing peers, while children with AS performed more poorly than typically developing controls. In this measure, the verbal content in the vignettes is masked; tone of voice is preserved but the lexical content cannot be determined. However, in identifying the nonverbal cues—such as facial expression, body language, and prosody—the NLD group had significantly more difficulty than the typically developing group, performing in a range consistent with the AS group. Thus, in a situation where verbal content is masked and the child must rely on nonverbal information alone in real-time interactions, children with NLD appeared to understand the interactions, but were not able to identify the nonverbal information shown as well as their typically developing peers (Semrud-Clikeman et al., 2014). Children with NLD were carefully screened for symptoms meeting the criteria for AS in this study, and the NLD diagnosis relied on both verbal/visual discrepancies and academic discrepancies.

Finally, in another study using the CASP video vignettes, children with a diagnosis of NLD *and* demonstrably poor social perception on the CASP also had more difficulty comprehending humor (e.g., cartoons, verbal nonsequiturs; Semrud-Clikeman & Glass, 2008; see Table 3.1). This finding was significant only

TABLE 3.1. Main Results of Selected Research Studies on Social and Emotional Difficulties in Children with NLD

Study	Social cue encoding/interpretation	Attention	Psychopathology
Dimitrovsky et al. (1998)	Interpretation of facial expressions: NLD < VLD and TD		
Worling et al. (1999)	Emotional inferencing: NLD < VLD and TD		
Petti et al. (2003)	Interpretation of facial expressions and gestures: NLD < VLD and TD		GLD/NLD > symptoms of depression than TD; no differences between NLD and GLD
Ralston et al. (2003)			Low-IQ children: mild internalizing had higher PIQs than more severe internalizing; no differences between groups in VIQ
Forrest (2004)			Internalized psychopathology: NLD = VLD = TD
Semrud-Clikeman & Glass (2010a, 2010b)	Humor comprehension: NLD = RD and TD; NLD + social difficulties < RD and TD		

50

Study			
Bloom & Heath (2010)	Recognition and understanding of facial expressions: GLD < NLD and TD	GLD > NLD/TD symptoms of inattention	Depression: GLD = NLD = TD
Semrud-Clikeman et al. (2010)	Evaluation of emotional cues: AS = NLD < ADHD and TD Evaluation of non-verbal cues: AS = NLD = ADHD < TD Social perception: AS = NLD < ADHD and TD	NLD and all other clinical groups symptoms > TD ADHD: C > other clinical groups	Depression: AS > TD; NLD > TD
Galway & Metsala (2011)	Evaluation of emotional and social cues: NLD < TD		
Semrud-Clikeman, Fine, & Bledsoe (2014)	Emotion recognition in video: NLD = TD Nonverbal cues in video: NLD = AS < TD		
Mammarella et al. (2015)			Generalized and social anxiety: NLD and RD > TD School and separation anxiety: NLD > TD Depression: RD > NLD and TD

Note. See Chapter 2 for more thorough discussion of the memory literature. NLD, nonverbal learning disability; RD, reading disability; VLD, verbal learning disability; GLD, general learning disability; AS, Asperger syndrome; ADHD, attention-deficit/hyperactivity disorder; TD, typically developing; VIQ, Verbal IQ; PIQ, Performance IQ.

when children with NLD who were low-performing on the CASP were compared with children with NLD who performed within a typical range on the CASP, indicating that not all children with NLD demonstrate functionally deficient social perception. The authors suggest that this may signal that there are subtypes of NLD with and without social perception deficits even though they all demonstrate visuospatial deficits. This study links social perception to other forms of social functioning for a subgroup of children with NLD. Notably, no differences in humor comprehension were found among all children with NLD in the study, children with reading disability (RD), and typically developing children. Thus, LD type may not be firmly tied to some aspects of social functioning, but rather dissociated and more dependent on basic social encoding and interpretation skills.

In summary, historically there is much anecdotal evidence for the idea that children with NLD might have more difficulty than other children with LD in the processing of social information. However, only a few studies have solidly confirmed this hypothesis empirically. Moreover, there is also evidence that problems in social functioning might be a global problem related to LD in general (Bauminger, Edelsztein, & Morash, 2005). Variation in research methods can make a big difference in results, as can the diagnostic criteria for who is enrolled in the studies. More careful research in this area is needed before the social information encoding issues specific to NLD can be understood. In addition, there may be other factors, such as attentional bias, that could influence how children with NLD perceive and encode social information.

Attention and Social Functioning

Attention is considered an important part of the social processing model not only because arousal to, and focus on, social cues has to occur before one can encode them, but later in the process as well. Crick and Dodge (1994) note that after encoding, arousal and focus are needed to select and plan for a desired goal (see Figure 3.1, step 3). This requires maintaining a mental representation of the current situation while formulating a plan,

drawing on previous experience, and holding the desired outcome in mind.

Problems with attention may influence encoding of social
cues at step 1 of the Crick and Dodge (1994) social processing
model. Looking at the literature on ASD, there is evidence that
some children focus on atypical areas of the face, such as the
mouth instead of the eyes, and on objects rather than faces,
and that these behaviors predict social competence (Klin, Jones,
Schultz, Volkmar, & Cohen, 2002). Verbal information has been
found to have more salience than visual information (Grossman,
Klin, Carter, & Volkmar, 2000), and behavioral inattention was
shown to account for variance in social perception in a sample of
children with HFA (Fine, Semrud-Clikeman, Butcher, & Walkowiak, 2008). Thus, from a clinical perspective, it is important to
consider whether inattention might influence a child's ability to
respond appropriately to social cues (see Table 3.1).

Only one study has evaluated attention in children with
NLD (Semrud-Clikeman et al., 2010b). Attention was measured
as a behavioral construct from the Structured Interview for Diagnostic Assessment of Children (SIDAC; Puig-Antich & Chambers, 1978), which identifies behavioral symptoms of inattention
consistent with the DSM-IV (American Psychiatric Association,
2000) diagnosis of ADHD, and from the attention scale of the
Behavioral Assessment System for Children–2 (BASC-2; Reynolds & Kamphaus, 2004). In this study, children with NLD were
identified based on low social skills, low mathematics scores relative to reasoning scores, and poor visuomotor integration. Children with NLD who met criteria for AS were moved to the AS
group. Typically developing controls and children with ADHD
were also included in the study. The results indicated that symptoms of inattention were related to perceiving nonverbal emotional cues on the CASP (Magill-Evans et al., 1995, 1996) but
not for recognition of emotional states of the actors in the video
vignettes. Behavioral symptoms of inattention in children with
NLD were found to be higher than typically developing controls,
but not significantly divergent from the AS; ADHD, inattentive;
or ADHD, combined, clinical groups.

In summary, it appears that inattention may be an important factor in social perception, particularly in recognizing the

nonverbal stream of information when interaction is naturalistic rather than static stimuli (e.g., photographs of faces). This is an area that needs further research, particularly with *in situ* or video stimuli. Notably, attentional symptoms appear to be present in NLD, and should be a part of a clinical evaluation of any child suspected of having an NLD profile. To date, no research has evaluated social processing in terms of sustained attention and complex tasks of WM.

Memory and Social Functioning

No study to date has evaluated the variation in social functioning or perception that might be accounted for by memory; thus, this is an area that is ready for further research. However, the consideration of NLD and of the associated mathematical disabilities suggests that the memory issue could be relevant. In particular, research literature in mathematics disability (MD) has indicated that WM deficits may be a part of the neuropsychological profile of MD (Alloway & Passolunghi, 2011; Bull & Scerif, 2001; Kyttälä, 2008; McLean & Hitch, 1999; Mabbot & Bisanz, 2008; Siegel & Ryan, 1989), but some studies have found no differences between mathematics skills and short-term and/or WM (e.g., Passolunghi & Siegel, 2001, 2004). Fletcher (1985) evaluated mode-specific memory (verbal vs. nonverbal) in children with language-based (reading and spelling) and arithmetic LD. He found that children with problems in arithmetic had more difficulty with nonverbal storage and retrieval for an abstract visuospatial dot-location memory task. Notably, the verbal memory task consisted of familiar words while the nonverbal task was novel and included no supporting context; thus, the memory tasks were not quite equivalent. It may be that had the list of words comprised novel or nonreal words, the outcome might have been different (Fletcher, 1985). However, more recent studies confirmed that children with MD have more difficulties in visuospatial than in verbal WM tasks (Passolunghi & Mammarella, 2010; Szucs, Devine, Soltesz, Nobes, & Gabriel, 2013).

As was covered in the previous chapter, there is evidence that children with NLD show particular problems with visuospatial WM, especially for complex tasks using the Corsi Block-Tapping

Task (e.g., Basso Garcia et al., 2014; Cornoldi et al., 2003; Mammarella & Cornoldi, 2005b). However, most of the research has focused on the relation between mathematics functioning and visuospatial memory.

Psychological Adjustment

As described above, most of the research on social functioning in NLD has looked at the ability to perceive and name emotions in faces and in video vignettes, as well as the subprocesses, such as attention, that may influence those skills. Although we tend to think that social skills are directly related to social *functioning*, there is little research that directly links social perception to social functioning and psychological adjustment directly in the NLD population. An important question to consider is whether children who have more difficulty perceiving social stimuli actually function more poorly socially. And if so, how might this affect long-term psychological adjustment?

The literature on LD shows that individuals with an LD, independent of the type of disability, may be at a greater risk for developing psychosocial disorders because they tend to have lower self-concepts, are less well socially accepted by their peers, and more anxious than children who do not have an LD (Howard & Tryon, 2002; Margalit & Shulman, 1986). However, whether a predisposition to internalizing disorders reflects a common biological pathway with LD or rather simple secondary and temporary consequences of the school failure remains unanswered. It is also important to note that the research on LD and psychopathology is quite variable, suggesting the influence of moderator variables such as gender, age, race, socioeconomic status, and whether samples are clinic or community based (Maag & Reid, 2006). Small and/or heterogeneous samples as well as differences in diagnostic methodology and methods may account for much of the variance in this literature (Fine et al., 2013). Moreover, differences observed may lack clinical and real-world meaning. For example, in their meta-analysis of depression in children, Maag and Reid (2006) found that although students with LD obtained higher depression scores than typically developing children, the degree of difference may not be sufficient to consider children with LD to be more at risk for a clinical affective disorder. Thus, when reviewing the literature on the psychological adjustment of children with NLD, attention to study samples, methods, and effect sizes is important. Another source of variability and ambiguity is represented by the outcome measures, which are usually rating scales of depressive and/or anxious symptoms. Rating scales can be designed for reporting either by the parent, teacher, or the child, and who does the reporting may also influence results (Youngstrom, Loeber, & Stouthamer-Loeber, 2000; Soma, Nakamura, Oyama, Tsuchiya, & Yamamoto, 2009).

Rating scales previously used with NLD are the PIC and the BASC, which are omnibus instruments designed to capture a variety of psychological symptoms. As discussed above, early on Rourke and his colleagues (e.g., Casey et al., 1991; Fuerst & Rourke, 1993; Rourke, 1989; Tsatsanis et al., 1997) reported that individuals with NLD are more likely than other persons to experience problems in psychological adjustment, particularly internalizing disorders, when using the PIC parent-reporting scale. Petti and coauthors (2003) also found that children with NLD were more likely to be diagnosed with an internalizing disorder than children with a verbal LD among children within a psychiatric treatment facility. However, in nonclinical community samples, this finding has not been easily replicated.

Within another clinical group, those with below-average IQ, Ralston, Fuerst, and Rourke (2003) replicated Fuerst et al. (1990) on psychopathology using the PIC described above. Raw counts of children classified as mild internalizing or more severe internalizing were analyzed on the basis of whether PIQ was greater or less than VIQ. Although there were no group differences in VIQ, those with PIQ lower than VIQ tended to sort into the more severe internalizing group. Group mean difference in PIQ was 6 standard scale points, but there were no data to show what the mean difference between VIQ and PIQ was within these low-functioning individuals, which makes the findings difficult to interpret and generalize.

Within community samples comprising children of at least average intellectual development, researchers using a variety of methods and diagnostic criteria for NLD have found that children with NLD are not more likely to experience problems in psychological adjustment than are their peers with verbal LD.

Forrest (2004) could not replicate psychopathology using parent reporting on the PIC, which was used in previous studies in Rourke's laboratory. Instead, children with a verbal LD were found to be at greater risk for withdrawal, while no differences between groups on any other internalizing psychopathology were observed based on parent ratings (Forrest, 2004).

Using the parent-report form of the BASC-2, Semrud-Clikeman and colleagues (2010b) found that children with AS, ADHD, or NLD as a broad clinical group, were more likely to be rated as having externalizing and internalizing symptoms compared with typically developing children. Specifically, children with NLD were rated as having more symptoms of depression than typically developing controls, but there were no differences between NLD and the other clinical groups; there were no differences between any clinical group and typically developing children on symptoms of anxiety; and children with NLD and AS both showed more symptoms of withdrawal than children with ADHD and typically developing controls. When teachers rather than parents reported, children with NLD were found to be no different from typically developing controls on the broad internalizing and externalizing factors, but the NLD group was found to have more anxiety symptoms than controls, similar to all of the other clinical groups. Thus, parents reported differently than teachers, with teachers indicating no differences specific to the NLD diagnosis.

Researchers using self-report of psychological adjustment have obtained varying results. Bloom and Heath (2010) found that adolescents with any type of LD endorsed more symptoms of depression than those without such challenges. However, no differences were found between the nonverbal and general LD groups. Using self-ratings from the BASC-2, Semrud-Clikeman et al. (2010b) found no differences between those with NLD and other clinical groups or typically developing controls on symptoms of social stress, anxiety, depression, or self-esteem. Those with HFA and ADHD, combined subtype, were found to have more social stress and depression than controls, while the ADHD, combined subtype, group had more symptoms of anxiety than controls. In contrast, Mammarella and Cornoldi (2014) did find some differences among children with NLD, those with RD, and neurotypical controls. Although both RD and NLD groups reported more general and social anxiety than the control group, children with NLD reported more symptoms of separation and school-related anxiety than children with no disability. Children with RD were found to report more depressive symptoms than those with NLD and typically developing controls. Mammarella and Cornoldi (2014) note that children with NLD may under-report internalized symptoms due to impaired emotional understanding, and further that the study was based on young children between ages 8 and 11, for whom depressive symptoms are less likely to manifest.

With such varying results within the research literature, it is difficult to conclusively determine whether the psychosocial adjustment of children with NLD differs from those with other types of LD. Further, the degree to which neurological substrates and/or environmental pressures associated with LD in general are most salient to psychopathology is quite unclear. For example, Antshel and Khan (2008) found an increase in certain psychiatric conditions in families including a child with NLD, and maternal stress related to dysfunctional interactions with the child was found to be increased in children with NLD (Antshel & Joseph, 2006). These findings have implications for psychosocial outcomes in NLD because parent involvement tends to predict psychosocial adjustment even better than academic achievement (El Nokali, Bachman, & Votruba-Drzal, 2010; Rueger, Malecki, & Demaray, 2010). If psychopathology is more evident in families with NLD, there may be both environmental and genetic contributions interacting to yield some children who have more severe social adjustment than others.

Semrud-Clikeman and Glass (2008), in fact, found two subgroups of NLD when evaluating humor: those with social deficits and those without. Others have also suggested that there may be subtypes of NLD that include or exclude various symptoms (e.g., Davis & Broitman, 2007; Forrest, 2004; Mamen, 2006; Palombo, 2006). For those with social deficits, this may be an important predictive factor for psychopathology; such children are more likely to be victimized by peers and siblings above the general population rates (Little, 2002). Thus, evaluation of the child with NLD should include an assessment of psychosocial functioning along with possible psychological and psychiatric sequelae.

Conclusions

This chapter highlighted the variation in findings for social perception and psychosocial adjustment in children with NLD. Most likely, findings are confounded by methodological, diagnostic, and developmental differences in the research. But just as likely, these variations reflect the wide range of heterogeneous symptoms present in the population we refer to as NLD. At the present state of the research we may conclude only that NLD, along with other types of LD, could be considered as a risk factor for developing psychosocial disorders. Thus, these variable findings serve as a reminder that each person should be treated as an individual with personal strengths and weaknesses requiring consideration not only in diagnosis but also in prognosis and intervention. Evaluating performance in visual, spatial, and verbal memory; attention; executive functioning; social perception; and psychosocial functioning should be part of any clinical characterization of a person with NLD.

CHAPTER FOUR

Neurological and Anatomical Evidence

Early Work on the Biological Bases of NLD

The neurodevelopmental basis of LD has long been recognized within the clinical literature. Early descriptions of individuals with RD made reference to a biological condition that produced an impairment in some area of the brain. Cases reported in the first half of the 20th century that were associated with learning difficulties were described as having a "brain dysfunction." The "minimal brain damage" profile described by Strauss and Lehtinen (1947) presented a variety of cognitive and behavioral impairments that also included weaknesses typical in NLD.

Early on, researchers describing neuropsychological profiles consistent with the NLD profile proposed a neurological model that implicated problems with right-hemisphere functioning. Although no mention was made of NLD, many studies reported descriptions of cognitive and social impairments thought to be associated with right-hemisphere functioning that largely overlapped with the NLD profile (Semrud-Clikeman & Hynd, 1990). For example, a study of children with right-hemisphere focal lesions showed that these children were particularly weak in spatial tasks (Stiles-Davis, Janowsky, Engel, & Nass, 1988). Stiles-Davis and colleagues reported on four children with congenital unilateral hemisphere injury and found that the two children with right-hemisphere injury were developmentally impaired in a copying task. In addition, their free drawings lacked configurational coherence; elements of the figures (e.g., the parts of a house) were present, but arrangement of the elements was spatially disorganized. Results were consistent with adult right-parietal brain injury functioning, who also demonstrated a similar failure in spatial organization. In contrast, the two children with left-hemisphere injury did not present any of these problems. Since the Stiles-Davis et al. report, an association between right-hemisphere lesions and difficulties in children's spatial cognition has been replicated in a series of studies. For example, Vicari, Stiles, Stern, and Resca (1998) found that children ages 3–5 with right-hemisphere injury performed significantly below children with left-hemisphere injury and typically developing controls on spatial construction tasks.

Evidence linking the right hemisphere to specific deficits was further extended to neurodevelopment in the absence of brain lesions. In the early 1980s, Weintraub and Mesulam (1983) first described patients with a developmental syndrome associated with right-hemisphere functioning. These children were characterized as having average intelligence and specific weaknesses in learning (especially in arithmetic), emotional and interpersonal difficulties, visuospatial disturbances, and inadequate paralinguistic communicative abilities. Similarly, Tranel et al. (1987) described a group of patients presenting neuropsychological evidence of right-hemisphere dysfunction, including severe deficits in nonverbal intelligence, visual memory, and visuospatial functions in the presence of high verbal skills. They concluded that this constellation of symptomatology represented a developmental LD of the right hemisphere. Evidence concerning this profile in children and their social weaknesses was then reported in a series of studies and reviewed by Semrud-Clikeman and Hynd (1990). Evidence concerning the association between the diagnosis of NLD and a right-hemisphere dysfunction was also reported by Nichelli and Venneri (1995), who studied a 22-year-old man with a developmental profile associated with arithmetic difficulties, visuospatial deficits, and emotional difficulties with intact language abilities. Through a PET scan they found a marked hypometabolism of the right hemisphere of the young man, thus supporting the claim that this type of LD is associated with functional abnormalities of the right hemisphere (see Figure 4.1).

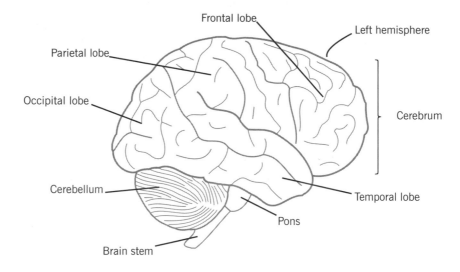

FIGURE 4.1. The human right hemisphere.

Reflection on the biological bases of the NLD profile was enriched by Rourke's early work as well. In 1987, Rourke introduced the "white-matter hypothesis," which highlighted the integrative nature of right-hemisphere tasks in comparison to left-hemispheric language-based tasks. Casey et al. (1991) reported on the Goldberg and Costa (1981) hypothesis (see also Goldberg, Vaughan, & Gerstman, 1978), which suggested that the right hemisphere has a greater ability to perform tasks requiring inter-modal integration, which is crucial for processing novel stimuli. In contrast, the left hemisphere was seen as important for uni-modal processing and storage; the model would predict a right-to-left shift in hemispheric dominance for the acquisition of new descriptive systems such as mathematics. Rourke extended the Goldberg and Costa hypothesis and theorized that differences in white-matter development in NLD may be the result of a pre-natal neuronal migration problem. He predicted that children with NLD, due to their neurological profile, would not make age-appropriate gains in problem solving, concept-formation abilities, hypothesis testing, and informational feedback. On this basis Rourke hypothesized a relative failure of children with NLD in making age-appropriate gains in visuoperceptual and problem-solving skills, mechanical arithmetic, and complex psychomotor and tactile–perceptual skills.

In his 1995 book, Rourke described major connective pathways (anterior–posterior, superior–inferior, right–left commissures) related with NLD, although he did not specify which of these pathways and how these pathways are presumed to be affected in children with NLD. In order to find evidence to test his psychobiological hypothesis, Rourke extended his research to children with genetic and medical conditions. In his most recent exposition of the white-matter hypothesis, Rourke, Rourke, and van der Vlugt (2002) identified neurological syndromes—such as AS, Turner syndrome, fetal alcohol syndrome, and traumatic brain injury—as disorders for which the phenotype is likely to include features of NLD. However, Spreen (2011), in his critical review of research on NLD, noted that not all children with such disorders show symptoms consistent with NLD, and some show symptoms that are not associated with NLD. Spreen (2011) and others (e.g., Filley, 2001, p. 262; c.f. Fine et al., 2013) have called for a more systematic program of neuroimaging work to identify the neural correlates of NLD that are linked to specific behavioral symptoms of the disorder.

Neuroimaging Research

Neuroimaging research on NLD is quite sparse, yet over the years the NLD profile of preserved verbal versus nonverbal skills has been associated with a variety of brain-based conditions including brain tumors (e.g., Carey, Barakat, Foley, Gyato, & Phillips, 2001), genetic disorders such as velocardiofacial syndrome (e.g., Lajiness-O'Neill et al., 2006), neurofibromatosis 1 (e.g., Varnhagen et al., 1988), Turner syndrome (e.g., Hong, Dunkin, & Reiss, 2011), and spina bifida (e.g., Ris et al., 2007), as well as prematurity (e.g., Grunau, Whitfield, & Davis, 2002). In these populations, researchers have observed problems in mathematics and social skills, visuospatial deficits, and discrepancies between verbal and nonverbal reasoning scores on standardized intelligence tests. However, many have also noted considerable individual variability in neuropsychological traits (e.g., Mazzocco, 2001;

Ris et al., 2007), indicating that caution is needed when applying an NLD heuristic to children who have neurological differences without careful clinical consideration. This is particularly salient to neuroimaging evidence because samples in these types of studies tend to be quite small, typically between five and 20 individuals per group. Individual characteristics can also influence results considerably.

In addition to a wide variance in individual characteristics and small samples, there are many other sources of error that can influence neuroimaging findings. Differences in experimental design and widely varying methods of analyses used to process very complex data (Weyandt, Swentosky, & Gudmundsdottir, 2013) have some neuroimaging experts concerned about overinterpretation of findings and the danger of establishing a modern phrenology (Karmiloff-Smith, 2010). The small body of neuroimaging work in NLD is no exception to these concerns. In its infancy, there has not been time for NLD findings to have been replicated, which is necessary for the scientific process to ensure some degree of reliability. Thus, the few studies presented below should be viewed with considerable caution.

Three neuroimaging studies that included a group of persons with NLD have been published to date. All of these studies have used the same pool of research participants, though each study does not include exactly the same sample due to matching and other considerations described below.

Presence of Cysts and Lesions

While scanning for a study on children with autism and NLD, researchers Semrud-Clikeman and Fine (2011) noticed that an unusually high number of children diagnosed with NLD showed benign cysts or legions of the brain. The study included 28 children with NLD, 26 with HFA (diagnosed as AS according to DSM-IV-TR criteria), and 24 typically developing controls. There were no differences in age (range 10–14 years) or Full Scale IQ among groups. Seven of the children in the NLD group were found to have a benign cyst or a lesion compared with one each in the HFA and typically developing groups. In the NLD group, three of the anomalies were located in the right hemisphere, three in the left, and one was a bilateral cerebellar cyst. For all but one of the children with NLD, the cysts/lesions were observed in the posterior regions of the brain.

Behaviorally, both the NLD and HFA groups demonstrated poorer social perception and visuomotor copy than the control group, but no significant differences between the HFA and NLD groups on these two measures were observed. Thus, special characteristics of the NLD group that could be related to the greater number of cysts/lesions were not observed except as determined by the diagnostic criteria for creating the clinical groups (e.g., mathematics skill, symptoms of autism). Therefore, interpreting these differences is not advised due to tautological problems. Finally, it is important to note that a consulting neuroradiologist read most of the cysts and lesions as benign, indicating that magnetic resonance imaging (MRI) is not automatically recommended for children with NLD unless there are other serious issues, loss of skill/functioning, or significant visuospatial problems that do not respond to intervention. However, the findings do suggest a possible neurodevelopmental difference in children with NLD compared with children with HFA and typically developing children.

Smaller Splenium of the Corpus Callosum

A further study (Fine, Musielak, & Semrud-Clikeman, 2014) examined the corpus callosum in children with NLD. The corpus callosum is a large white-matter tract connecting the right and left hemispheres of the brain. The splenium is the posterior aspect of the corpus callosum, comprising fibers that serve the posterior temporal, parietal, and occipital regions of the brain (see Figure 4.2). Thus the primary and secondary visual areas as well as associative regions merging visual, language, and spatial/sensory functions are connected via the posterior portion of the corpus callosum.

Nineteen children with NLD; 23 with HFA (diagnosed as AS with DSM-IV-TR criteria); 23 with ADHD, combined type; 25 with ADHD, inattentive type; and 57 neurotypical controls were included in the study. Children with midline cysts were excluded. There were no differences among groups in Full Scale IQ. Measurements of the corpus callosum were calculated as area of the structure at the midline where it crosses between hemispheres, and the effect of whole-brain size calculated as midline area of the cerebrum was removed via regression. Age was controlled for in all analyses. In this study, children with NLD were found to have significantly smaller areas of the splenium compared with other groups. Within the NLD group, those with smaller splenium size performed more poorly on the Weschler Abbreviated Scale of Intelligence (WASI; Wechsler, 1999) PIQ, whereas this association was not observed in the HFA group. No relation between splenium size and VIQ was observed in either group.

These findings lend support to the proposition set out by Rourke years ago (e.g., Harnadek & Rourke, 1994; Rourke, 1995) that NLD is a disorder of visuospatial processing by demonstrating an observable anatomical difference in the visuospatial system that is also associated with differences in visuospatial reasoning. These findings also suggest that this anatomical difference may be unique to children with NLD, and not associated with HFA. However, it must be noted that the groups in this study were small, and the findings have not been validated in other samples. Just as recent advances in autism have demonstrated that the spectrum comprises heterogeneous genetic pathways to a common phenotype, NLD may also be considerably diverse—thus a few individuals may easily influence results.

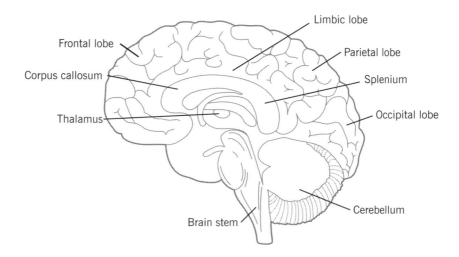

FIGURE 4.2. A midsagittal view showing the inner boundaries of the lobes of the cerebral cortex.

Neuroanatomical Similarities to Autism in Social Structures

As discussed in previous chapters, there are some overlapping behavioral characteristics in NLD and HFA, particularly the subgroup referred to above as having AS. Difficulty with social relationships as well as problems when presented with novel environments or tasks (Semrud-Clikeman & Fine, 2011) are among the similarities between these two groups. In contrast, children with NLD do not seem to present with intense narrow interests or stereotypic repetitive behaviors (Broitman & Davis, 2013). Although some children with autism may have deficits in visuospatial functioning, this trait is not ubiquitous in autism. Thus, it is in the neural systems related to social functioning where anatomical similarities might be observed between the groups, particularly if the overlap in social symptoms develops via similar neurodevelopmental progressions. On the other hand, if social difficulties arise from differing etiological processes, then one might expect differences between groups in the social networks of the brain.

Several anatomical structures that are involved in the social circuitry of the brain have been identified; most of these are subcortical structures located toward the center of the brain and are considered to be part of broad neural circuitries. The amygdalae have long been associated with emotional processing and emotional learning—particularly important in early processing of strong salient emotions from the environment, positive or negative, the amygdalae are implicated in emotional biographical memories (Staniloiu & Markowitsch, 2012). In autism, these structures have been found to be larger, although not consistently so (see Bauman & Kemper, 2005, for a review); age may be a factor with differences showing in younger groups but not older (Stanfield et al., 2008). The hippocampus is another structure implicated in autism—this subcortical structure, occurring bilaterally like the amygdala, is also involved in memory of biographical events and has been found to be larger in some studies, but quite inconsistently (Stanfield et al., 2008). The caudate nucleus has been consistently observed as larger in autism (Stanfield et al., 2008) but has not been studied in children with HFA for whom anatomical differences may be different from typically developing children (Semrud-Clikeman, Fine, Bledsoe, & Zhu,

2013). The caudate has been implicated in memory, social behavior, and learning, particularly in goal-directed motor movement (Grahn, Parkinson, & Owen, 2008). Finally, the anterior cingulate cortex, which is a portion of the cortex overlying the subcortical structures discussed above that is positioned nearest to the frontal lobes, is thought to be related to attention and orienting in relation to emotion processing (Etkin, Egner, & Kalisch, 2011). This region has not been well studied in HFA (Semrud-Clikeman et al., 2013), and none of the structures above had been evaluated in NLD until the study carried out by Semrud-Clikeman and colleagues, described below.

In a study sample that included 29 children with NLD, 29 with HFA (diagnosed as AS with DSM-IV-TR criteria), and 31 typically developing controls, no differences were found in total brain volume, total white matter, or total gray matter of the brain among groups. Differences in age and VIQ were not significant. The study showed that children with NLD had volumes similar to that of the typically developing controls for both the left and right amygdalae, as well as the left and right hippocampi. The HFA group had significantly larger volumes than both the control and NLD groups bilaterally for the amygdalae and hippocampi. Both the HFA and NLD groups had smaller volumes in both the left and right anterior cingulate cortex. No differences among groups were observed in the caudate.

Previous findings of enlarged brain structures in autism (Stanfield et al., 2008) were partially replicated in this study, particularly in the reciprocally connected amygdalar–hippocampal network (Groen, Teluj, Buitelaar, & Tendolkar, 2010). Notably, children with NLD did not show evidence of this abnormality, which is thought to be related to aberrant neuronal development and pruning. The anterior cingulate finding, for which both the HFA and NLD groups showed reduced volumes compared with controls, may suggest underdevelopment of a region involved in regulating the activation of the amygdala during emotional conflict (Etkin, Prater, Hoeft, Menon, & Schatzberg, 2014).

One limitation of this study is that the volumetric findings were not related to behavioral characteristics. Thus, it is difficult to extrapolate how these differences manifest functionally, if at all. However, the study does give first evidence that children with NLD may have the aberrant connectivity seen in those with autism, particularly with respect to enlargement of subcortical structures.

Conclusions

The neuroanatomical evidence for NLD is just emerging. There are so few studies, and none replicated, that little can be reliably drawn from the work. So far, the extant research seems to support a visuospatial hypothesis, and also seems to show distinction for NLD with respect to autism. Children with NLD and HFA may demonstrate some similar behavioral features, but from a neurodevelopmental perspective based on these few studies, NLD brains do not strongly resemble those with autism.

In the future, multiple methods must converge to verify the neural processes involved in NLD and should include more than neuroimaging only. Rather, researchers need to begin tying neuroimaging findings directly to behaviors, genetics, and environmental factors that could be involved in shaping the neuropsychological characteristics associated with NLD. Some researchers have found that siblings of children with NLD profiles who have an associated genetic disorder also show signs of NLD (e.g., Cutting, Koth, & Denckla, 2000; Lajiness-O'Neill et al., 2006). Since not *all* children with specific genetic disorders show the profile, it may be that NLD is a familial developmental pattern independent of other brain disturbances, including autism. Sibling studies describing familial differences in neuroanatomy and function using functional magnetic resonance imaging may also provide an important research methodology in the future.

CHAPTER FIVE

The Diagnostic Criteria

Looking for a Consensus

International comparisons have shown that even when the existence of a specific disorder is well accepted, as in the cases of dyslexia and dyscalculia, identification criteria, cutoffs, and provisions of the diagnosis may substantially vary (Al-Yagon et al., 2013). Consequently, epidemiological and research data, policies, and evidence-based treatments are biased by the specific procedures adopted in the different contexts. In this respect, it may not be surprising that the NLD diagnosis encompasses a certain degree of variability. However, in the case of NLD, the problem is more serious because the existence of the disorder is debated. Fifty years from its first description there is still no consensus on the criteria for diagnosing children with NLD nor on the merits of identifying it as a specific disorder; not only is this disorder absent from the clinical classification systems but the related research and practice have not been adequately developed.

To the present day, the procedures for detecting the core features of NLD have not been clearly established (Ris & Nortz, 2008)—thus, researchers find it difficult to define the NLD samples in their research. Moreover, a lack of consensus as to what the "disability" refers (e.g., mathematics, visuospatial, social perception, deficits, or some combination of any or all of these characteristics), has impeded forward progress in establishing well-founded diagnostic procedures and prognostic information to parents and clinicians.

Typical Criteria Used by Clinicians for Making a Diagnosis of NLD

Despite the lack of a full consensus, the diagnosis of NLD is rather frequent, either alone or in association with another diagnosis recognized by the most popular diagnostic manuals. Actually, some form of diagnosis appears necessary in order to help these children. As Fine and colleagues (Fine, Semrud-Clikeman, Bledsoe, & Musielak, 2013) recently stated:

> We empathize with neuropsychologists and psychologists who must apply a label to children in order to obtain payment and/or services. Currently, describing a child as having NLD yields weak empirical links to intervention (Fletcher & Dennis, 2010), but may nonetheless be the best option for a child who is struggling but otherwise does not fit extant DSM or educational diagnostic criteria. We encourage clinicians to do what they already do best, to describe the characteristics of children in a way that helps them succeed in the world. (p. 30)

The results of Solodow and coauthors' (2006) survey, reported in Chapter 1, showed that many clinicians use the NLD diagnosis and, on many points, share the same views. The diagnosis has been inspired by the symptom descriptions offered in the pioneering work of Johnson and Myklebust (1967) and Rourke (1989), reviewed in Chapter 1, and subsequently developed by clinicians working in various countries. Specifically, the early conceptualization of NLD made by Rourke arose from the differentiation of language- versus arithmetic-based learning problems. In fact, Rourke's early studies required that children identified with NLD only show poor arithmetic scores (Rourke & Finlayson, 1978; Rourke & Strang, 1978). Over time, the criteria have changed (see Table 5.1), becoming more specific, less concerned with the area of LD, and evolving to reflect the neuropsychological assets and deficits hypothesized to characterize children with NLD according to Rourke's (1989) model.

TABLE 5.1. Historical Development of Diagnostic Criteria for NLD Made by Rourke and Collaborators

Rourke & Finlayson (1978); Rourke & Strang (1978)	Strang & Rourke (1983)	Harnadek & Rourke (1994)	Pelletier, Ahmad, & Rourke (2001); Drummond, Ahmad & Rourke (2005)
• WRAT Arithmetic > 1.8 below grade	• WRAT Reading/ Spelling > WRAT Arithmetic by 2 years	• WISC VIQ > 79 • VIQ > PIQ (10 points) • WRAT Reading/ Spelling > Arithmetic (10 points) • Speech-Sounds Perception or Auditory Closure < 1 *SD* below mean • Target Test > 1 *SD* below mean • Grooved Pegboard > 1 *SD* below mean (either hand) • Dysgraphesthesia or finger agnosia or astereognosis > 1 *SD* below mean	First five or seven or more of eight below: 1. Target Test 1 *SD* below mean 2. Finger agnosia/ dysgraphia/ astereognosis composite > 1 *SD* below mean *and* less than two errors on tactile perception 3. The WISC subtests U, S, I are highest of the Verbal Scale 4. The WISC subtests BD, OA, and Coding are lowest of the Performance Scale 5. WRAT Reading > Arithmetic (8 points) 6. Tactile performance test right > left > both 7. Grip strength within 1 *SD* of mean *and* Grooved Pegboard > 1 *SD* below mean 8. WISC VIQ > PIQ (10 points)

Note. Based on Fine, Semrud-Clikeman, Bledsoe, and Musielak (2013). WRAT, Wide Range Achievement Test; WISC, Wechsler Intelligence Scale for Children; VIQ, Verbal IQ; PIQ, Performance IQ; *SD*, Standard Deviation; V, Vocabulary; S, Similarities; I, Information; BD, Block Design; OA, Object Assembly.

In particular, Pelletier, Ahmad, and Rourke (2001) and Drummond et al. (2005) tried to define the criteria for diagnosing children with NLD for 9- to 15-year-olds and 7- to 8-year-olds, respectively. Their criteria for young children mentioned the following points: (1) tactile perception impairments, (2) reading better than mathematical achievement, (3) at least two of the following subtests on the WISC (Wechsler, 1974, 1991) available at that time—Vocabulary, Similarities, and Information—obtain the highest results on the Verbal scale, (4) at least two WISC subtests—Block Design, Object Assembly, and Coding—obtain the lowest results on the Performance scale, (5) poor visuoconstructive skills, (6) motor-coordination impairments, (7) tactile performance impairments, and (8) a VIQ at least 10 points higher than the PIQ on the WISC. For the older children (ages 9–15), five or six of these traits meant a likely diagnosis of NLD, while for the younger ones (ages 7–8), three criteria were considered sufficient for the diagnosis: visuoconstructive impairments and specific patterns in the subtests on the Verbal and Performance scales in the WISC (criteria 3 and 4 above). Table 5.1 summarizes the development of diagnostic criteria for NLD according to Rourke and coworkers (2001, 2005). In the last column we report the latest-to-date proposed criteria, in which the authors also cited the tests recommended for the diagnosis.

One limitation of Rourke's diagnostic criteria is that, being related to specific tests, the diagnoses may become obsolete when new versions of tests are published. For example, VIQs and PIQs are not considered in the most recent versions of the WISC, particularly in the versions most largely used at this time (WISC-IV and -V; Wechsler, 2003, 2014), in which at least four factorial indices and total IQ can be computed; the Verbal and Perceptual indexes only partly reflect the old indexes. In addition, some criteria were not justified—for example, the 10-point discrepancy between VIP and PIQ (Pelletier et al., 2001) is neither significant nor rare among well-functioning children.

Recent Reviews of the Literature

There has been a remarkable effort among researchers to identify and treat a group of children who struggle with visuospatial, academic, and social problems during the past three decades. Rourke and his colleagues (2001, 2005), in particular, have established the most detailed descriptions of children who fit the NLD profile, but changes in research methods, including greater efforts at internal and external validation, are required for the field to move forward. Specifically, attention to issues of diagnostic criteria, exclusion or recognition of comorbid influences, consensus on the role of social deficits, and differentiation in relation to typically developing children are all research issues needing attention. A substantial consensus is needed in research in order to compare the results of different studies that are based on the assumption that they concern the same population. A review of the scientific literature referring to children with NLD may clarify the issue of the identification criteria. Table 5.2 summarizes the diagnostic criteria for children with NLD used in peer-reviewed papers published from 1985 to 2015. The present review is partly based on two previous reviews (Fine et al., 2013; Mammarella & Cornoldi, 2014) we coauthored.

In 2013, Fine et al. published a critical review of the literature on NLD and defined the following conditions for including research studies in their review:

- Adequate sample description.
- Presence of a control group with typical development.
- Quantitatively defined diagnostic criteria.
- Exclusion of comorbid medical/neurological diagnoses.
- Sample sizes appropriate for method used.
- Absence of tautological problems.

Based on their research on publications between January 1975 and March 2010 they found 63 peer-reviewed publications excluding dissertations and theses, but when studies with no statistical analyses of dependent variables were excluded, only 32 publications remained.

The diagnostic criteria used to define the NLD groups in the peer-reviewed publications analyzed by Fine and coauthors (2013) appear to align with the broader conceptualization of NLD advanced by Rourke and colleagues (2001, 2005) with few exceptions. Stronger reading than mathematics skills were fairly consistently used: reading was most often measured by the WRAT

(Jastak & Jastak, 1965) or the Wechsler Individual Achievement Test (WIAT; Breaux, 2009); discrepancies between reading and math were widely found, with the number of points of discrepancy ranging from 8 to 15. Differences in VIQ and nonverbal PIQ measures were widely found among the studies. Only eight did not include VIQ > PIQ as a criterion. Although tactile and motor deficits were considered in Rourke's (1989) model to be a primary deficit, many studies did not include this as part of the diagnostic criteria for NLD group inclusion. Similarly, while the conceptualization of visual and visuomotor deficits was posited as central to the NLD syndrome, very few studies included a measure of these skills. Finally, social deficits were simply noted as "poor" or noted by qualitative features, such as "paralinguistic problems."

The review of the literature by Fine and coauthors (2013) observed that many of the peer-reviewed studies of NLD included more than one methodological problem. Of the 32 studies reviewed, around 19% met all of the research conditions reported above, 34% met all but one condition, and the remaining 47% failed to meet two or more of the conditions outlined for this review. Of those examined, the conditions most frequently violated were failure to include a typically developing control group (around 56%), failure to provide adequate exclusionary criteria (around 52%), and the use of no quantitatively defined diagnostic criteria (around 28%). Most studies (around 94%) reported at least the gender and age of their participants, but more than half (around 55%) reported neither ethnicity nor socioeconomic status. Half of the studies included sample sizes with 15 or fewer participants in the NLD group (around 45%). In conclusion, the review of the literature revealed that of the 32 studies examined, only six had all of the characteristics of methodology expected in modern empirical work according to the authors. Thus, Fine and coauthors concluded that the historical research on NLD may be poorly reliable due to small sample sizes, lack of exclusionary criteria, vague sample descriptions, and poor attention to comorbid conditions that do not allow generalization of the research findings.

In another recent review, Mammarella and Cornoldi (2014) analyzed which identification criteria were most often used in the scientific literature on NLD and which variables best

TABLE 5.2. Diagnostic Criteria Used by Researchers to Diagnose Children with NLD

Study	Verbal vs. nonverbal intelligence discrepancy	Visuoconstructive and fine-motor impairment	VSWM impairment	Reading vs. mathematics discrepancy	Social skills
Tranel et al. (1987)	From 13 to 38 points	Low scores on the Rey Complex Figure Test	Low scores on the Benton Visual Retention Test (1974)	Good reading achievement and poor math achievement	Low social and emotional abilities
Casey et al. (1991)	VIQ > PIQ (10 points)	Low scores on the Target Test and on the Grooved Pegboard Test		Reading > math (10 points)	
Harnadek & Rourke (1994)	VIQ > PIQ (10 points)	Low scores on the Target Test and on the Grooved Pegboard Test	Low scores on the Tactual Perceptual Test–Memory and Location	Reading > math (10 points)	
Gross-Tsur et al. (1995)	VIQ > PIQ and VIQ > 85	Soft neurological signs on the left side of the body		Math achievement 1 year below class level	Emotional and interpersonal behavioral disorders
Cornoldi et al. (1995)	Verbal intelligence > spatial intelligence			Poor math achievement	

Study	IQ criteria	Neuropsychological/motor	Cognitive/memory	Academic	Social/emotional
Fisher & DeLuca (1997)	9 points and VIQ > 79	Low scores on the Target Test and on the Grooved Pegboard Test		Reading > math (10 points)	
Fisher et al. (1997)	VIQ > PIQ (9 points) and VIQ > 79	Low scores on the Target Test and on the Grooved Pegboard Test		Reading > math (10 points)	
Dimitrovsky et al. (1998)			z-scores < 0 on the Benton Visual Retention test (1974)		
Cornoldi et al. (1999)	VIQ > PIQ (15 points)	Poor handwriting	Low scores on VSWM tasks	Poor math achievement	Low social abilities
Worling et al. (1999)	VIQ > PIQ (10 points); VIQ > 85 and PIQ < 85			Math < reading; math < 25th percentile	
Chow & Skuy (1999)	VIQ > PIQ (15 points)	Poor visuomotor integration and fine-motor coordination	Visuospatial and organizational problems	Reading > math; reading decoding > reading comprehension	Poor socioemotional functioning

(continued)

TABLE 5.2. (continued)

Study	Verbal vs. nonverbal intelligence discrepancy	Visuoconstructive and fine-motor impairment	VSWM impairment	Reading vs. mathematics discrepancy	Social skills
Pelletier et al. (2001)	VIQ > PIQ (10 points); (a) Two of WISC PIQ scale: OA, BD, and Coding subtests score lowest; (b) two of WISC VIQ scale: V, S, I subtests score highest	Low scores on the Target Test and on the Grooved Pegboard Tactual Performance Tests		Reading > math (8 points)	
Petti et al. (2003)	12 points			Math 1 SD lower than VIQ	
Venneri et al. (2003)	V > BD		Low scores on VSWM tasks	> 30th percentile	
Forrest (2004)	VCI > POI (12 points) (WISC)	Low scores on the Target Test and on the Grooved Pegboard Test		Reading > math (8 points)	
Humphries et al. (2004)	VIQ > PIQ (10 points)			Reading > math (10 points); math < 25th percentile	

Study					
Drummond et al. (2005)	VIQ > PIQ (10 points); see Pelletier et al. (2001)	Low scores on the Target Test and on the Grooved Pegboard Test	Reading > math (8 points)	Low scores on the Child Behavior Checklist	
Liddell & Rasmussen (2005)	10 points; see Pelletier et al. (2001)		Low scores on visual memory	Reading > math; reading decoding > reading comprehension	
Mammarella & Cornoldi (2005a)	Verbal intelligence > spatial intelligence		Low scores on VSWM tasks		
Mammarella & Cornoldi (2005b)	VIQ > PIQ (10 points)		Low scores on VSWM tasks		
Yu et al. (2006)				Math lower than predicted	
Antshel & Joseph (2006)		Impaired visuospatial and motor abilities		Reading > math	Poor social interaction

(continued)

TABLE 5.2. (continued)

Study	Verbal vs. nonverbal intelligence discrepancy	Visuoconstructive and fine-motor impairment	VSWM impairment	Reading vs. mathematics discrepancy	Social skills
Hendriksen et al. (2007)	VIQ > PIQ (10 points); see Pelletier et al. (2001)	Low scores on the VMI		Reading > math	
Semrud-Clikeman & Glass (2008)	V > BD (WISC)	Low scores on the VMI, JLO, and Rey Complex Figure Test	Reading ≥ 85; math below average		
Antshel & Khan (2008)		Impaired visuospatial abilities; motor coordination more marked in the left side		Well-developed reading and poor mechanical arithmetic	Deficits in social perception, judgment, and interaction
Schiff et al. (2009)		Low scores on the Benton Visual Retention Test (1974)	Low scores on the Benton Visual Retention Test (1974)	Poor math achievement	

Study				
Mammarella et al. (2009)	VIQ > PIQ (10 points); see Pelletier et al. (2001)		Reading > 50th percentile	
Semrud-Clikeman et al. (2010a)	Vocabulary > 85 (WISC)	Low scores on the VMI, Rey Complex Figure Test, and Purdue Pegboard Test (Tiffin, 1968)	Reading > 50th percentile; math < 15th percentile	Low scores on the Social Skills Rating Scale
Semrud-Clikeman et al. (2010b)	Vocabulary > 85 (WISC)	Low scores on the VMI and the Purdue Pegboard Test	1 SD lower than IQ	Low scores on the Social Skills Rating Scale
Grodzinsky et al. (2010)	VIQ > PIQ (10 points); VCI > POI (10 points) (WISC)	Low scores on the Grooved Pegboard Test		Reading > math
Bloom & Heath (2010)			Reading > 85; math < 80	
Mammarella et al. (2010a)		Low scores on VSWM tasks	Reading > 50th percentile and poor math achievement	

(continued)

TABLE 5.2. (continued)

Study	Verbal vs. nonverbal intelligence discrepancy	Visuoconstructive and fine-motor impairment	VSWM impairment	Reading vs. mathematics discrepancy	Social skills
Mammarella & Pazzaglia (2010)	Verbal intelligence > spatial intelligence	Low scores on the Target Test	Low scores on VSWM tasks	> 50th percentile	
Galway & Metsala (2011)	VIQ > PIQ (10 points)	< 25th percentile in handwriting skills and on the Grooved Pegboard Test		Reading > 30th percentile; math < 25th percentile	
Lepach & Petermann (2011)	VIQ > PIQ	Low scores on drawing tasks			
Mammarella et al. (2013a)	VIQ > PIQ (15 points); VCI > POI	VMI < 30th percentile		Average performance for speed and/or accuracy on reading; math < 1 SD on two of three tasks	

Semrud-Clikeman et al. (2013)	VIQ > 85	Rey Complex Figure Test scores < 1 *SD*; Purdue Pegboard Test scores < 1 *SD*	Math skills < 15th percentile; math skills < 1.5 *SD* than FSIQ	Nonverbal score on the CASP test < 1 *SD*; social skills (Vineland Adaptive Behavior Scale) < 85
Basso Garcia et al. (2014)	Low scores on BD; nonverbal intelligence < 1.5 *SD*	Low scores on the Rey Complex Figure Test	Average reading	
Semrud-Clikeman et al. (2014)	VIQ > 85; low scores on BD	Rey Complex Figure Test scores < 1 *SD*; Purdue Pegboard Test scores < 1 *SD*	Math skills < 15th percentile; math skills < 1.5 *SD* than FSIQ	Nonverbal score on the CASP test < 1 *SD*; social skills (Vineland Adaptive Behavior Scale) < 85
Mammarella et al. (2015)	VIQ > PIQ (15 points); VCI > POI	VMI Test < 30th percentile	Average performance for speed and/or accuracy on reading	

Note. VSWM, Visuospatial Working Memory; VIQ, Verbal IQ; PIQ, Performance IQ; WISC, Wechsler Intelligence Scale for Children; OA, Object Assembly; BD, Block Design; V, Vocabulary; S, Similarities; I, Information; *SD*, Standard Deviation; VMI, Visual–MotorIntegration Test; JLO, Judgment of Line Orientation; FSIQ, Full Scale IQ; CASP, Child and Adolescent Social Perception; VCI, Verbal Comprehension Index; POI, Perceptual Organization Index.

distinguished children with NLD from typically developing controls. The classic effect size index (*d*) proposed by Cohen (1988) was calculated to establish the magnitude of differences identified. This index was used for describing the mean standardized difference between children with NLD and typically developing controls. For example, a *d* value of 0.5 indicated that the mean value in the NLD group for a particular selection criterion differed from the value found in a control group or another clinical group by half a standard deviation, corresponding to a medium effect size. Cohen's *d* was calculated for two kinds of variables: (1) variables used as internal criteria for selecting children with NLD (e.g., VIQ and PIQ, visuoconstructive and fine-motor skills, achievement in reading and mathematics), and (2) dependent variables (mainly visuospatial memory, emotion comprehension, social skills) examined in groups of children with a diagnosis of NLD given without referring to those aspects.

Searching publications from January 1980 to February 2012, Mammarella and Cornoldi (2014) initially found 66 publications in English. The requisites of a study to be included in the review were the mention of the criteria adopted to select children with NLD and the quantitative data. In addition, only publications in which a group of children with NLD was compared with a group of typically developing controls and/or another clinical group were included. Using this procedure, 35 papers were identified.

The main results of the review showed that the two most frequently adopted criteria were, first, the consideration of VIQ and nonverbal or visuospatial IQ (28 studies), either separately or as a discrepancy measure; and, second, the consideration of achievement in reading and mathematics (31 studies), again either separately or as a discrepancy measure. Visuoconstructive and motor-coordination deficits were often considered as well (in 20 and 15 studies, respectively). As expected there was a substantial difference in the effect size between the variables used as diagnostic criteria and outcome variables. In short, combining the results obtained with the variables used as internal criteria with those considered as dependent variables, the strongest criteria for selecting children with NLD were visuospatial intelligence and the discrepancy between VIQ and visuospatial intelligence. It is noteworthy that a Cohen's *d* = 1 would correspond to a difference of 15 points in the traditional IQ measures, and that the analyses revealed group differences substantially higher than 1.5 standard deviations from the mean (i.e., corresponding to more than 22 standardized IQ points). Visuoconstructive and fine-motor skills, discrepancy between mathematics and reading achievement, and mathematics achievement and spatial memory were also associated with high effect sizes, while visuospatial memory and socioemotional skills revealed a medium effect size. Finally, the lowest values were observed for verbal intelligence, visual memory, and reading achievement, for which there was no substantial mean difference between the NLD and control groups.

Proposed Diagnostic Criteria for NLD

Based on the reviews made by Fine et al. (2013) and Mammarella and Cornoldi (2014), we propose inclusion and exclusion criteria for diagnosing children with NLD, though we are well aware that this is only a starting point on the path toward a consensus among researchers. Inclusion criteria make reference to five main points; exclusion criteria are defined as well. The criteria are presented here, with commentary following.

- *Criterion A*. A persistent deficit in one or more measures of nonverbal intelligence or reasoning (e.g., perceptual reasoning, visuospatial intelligence) in the presence of an average or above-average verbal intelligence.
- *Criterion B*. Substantial weaknesses, currently or emerging from the child's history, in processing visuospatial information, as manifested by at least two of the following weaknesses:
    1. Difficulties in perceiving organized forms (e.g., extreme difficulties in the analysis and recognition of gestalts).
    2. Difficulties in reproducing simple drawings by copy or memory (e.g., extreme difficulties in copying simple geometrical figures, or complex figures in visuoconstructive tasks).
    3. Difficulties in temporarily remembering and manipu-

lating visuospatial information (e.g., low scores in visuo-spatial short-term memory or visuospatial WM tasks).

• *Criterion C.* Presence of clinical and/or psychometric indexes of weaknesses in at least one of the following areas, currently or by history:

1. Fine-motor impairments including praxis and/or output (e.g., in using hands for drawing or handwriting; in using zippers, fastening buttons, tying shoelaces when dressing).
2. Poor academic achievement in activities involving visuo-spatial skills, mathematics, or other, in the presence of an average or above-average performance in reading decoding tasks (e.g., difficulties in writing numbers; visuospatial errors in written calculations, such as column confusion, carrying/borrowing errors; difficulties with mirrored numbers, geometry, comprehension of visuospatial relationships and descriptions, interpreting graphs and tables).
3. Difficulties in social interactions (e.g., verbose speaking; difficulties in understanding nonverbal communication, interpreting facial expressions).

• *Criterion D.* Several symptoms were present before age 7, although they could not have become fully manifest until academic demands exceeded children's capacities, or were masked by good verbal strategies.

• *Criterion E.* There is clear evidence that the symptoms interfere with, or reduce the quality of, academic, occupational, or social functioning.

• *Criterion F.* These disorders are not better explained by the presence of ASD or DCD. The diagnosis of NLD can be given in the presence of the "soft" symptoms of ASD or DCD, but if the criteria for those disorders are met, the diagnosis of NLD does not apply. Similarly, if the NLD profile seems a consequence of a condition of intellectual disability, sensory disabilities, neurological, and/or genetic conditions, the diagnosis of NLD is not applied. However, in all these cases, the diagnosis will mention the fact that the child presents symptoms consistent with an NLD profile.

Diagnostic Features
of the First Three Proposed Criteria

An essential feature of NLD is a persistent deficit in nonverbal intelligence in the presence of an average or above-average verbal intelligence. Historically, Rourke (1995) proposed a discrepancy of at least 10 points between WISC VIQ and PIQ, but this criterion seems too weak as it fails to reflect a statistically significant departure from the population-based normative data obtained with the WISC (Wechsler, 1974, 1991). In addition, the latest versions of the WISC do not allow for the calculation of VIQ and PIQ; only factorial indices can be calculated and the focus is on more specific verbal and visuospatial (perceptual) indexes. Furthermore, the referral to a single intelligence battery may create problems for clinicians who used different tests for measuring general cognitive abilities.

We therefore suggest that the criterion makes a more general reference to relatively pure measures of verbal and perceptual/ visuospatial intelligence. These measures would be obtained with a battery of intellectual subtests when a perceptual/visuospatial intelligence weakness is mentioned in the presence of an average or above-average verbal intelligence, with the consequence of a discrepancy between the two areas of intelligence (e.g., a marked discrepancy between the visuoconstructive and Perceptual Organization Index/Perceptual Reasoning Index (POI/PRI) factorial indices of the WISC). This criterion has typically been adopted for a diagnosis of NLD, although its exact definition seems to be debatable. Among the problems related with this criterion are the vagueness of the underlying model of intelligence and the weakness of a discrepancy criterion. In fact, within the diagnostic criteria for the corresponding verbal disorders (e.g., language disorder, specific reading LD) the Verbal Intelligence Index is not required to be particularly low. These issues are now also a focus of debate within the field of intelligence—for example, it is argued that pure measures of visuospatial and verbal intelligence may be made more independent from general measures of intelligence. In any case, concerning a discrepancy between verbal and nonverbal intelligence, we notice that for a discrepancy to be meaningful it should be considerably large (e.g., at least one standard deviation). However, we think that the main focus should be on poor perceptual/visuospatial intelligence in the presence of good verbal intelligence, rather than on the discrepancy per se. In fact, the criterion should not be applied to cases with discrepancies in the highest or lowest IQ ranges. In particular, when a very high verbal intelligence is associated with an adequate visuospatial intelligence score (not due to the use of compensating verbal strategies) and there is no corroborating evidence that the symptoms interfere with academic, occupational, or social functioning, the diagnosis is not warranted. In contrast, when a low verbal intelligence (e.g., < 85) is associated with a very poor visuospatial intelligence the diagnosis of NLD should be given cautiously and alternative diagnoses should be taken into consideration.

The second criterion refers to weaknesses in processing visuospatial information, specifically, poor performance in visual perception, visuospatial short-term memory or WM, and visuoconstructive tasks. It is worth noting that visuospatial memory was not historically considered as a possible criterion for selecting children with NLD, but the review of the scientific literature and the clinical evidence showed a substantial impairment in visuospatial memory performance between children with NLD and typically developing controls (Mammarella & Cornoldi, 2014). We suggest using more than a task for assessing visuospatial memory in order to have a clear picture of the child's functioning. Similarly, we recommend obtaining more than one measure of visuoconstructive skills—for example, using both the VMI (Beery & Buktenica, 2006) and the Rey–Osterrieth Complex Figure (ROCF; Osterrieth, 1944), and obtaining in at least one measure a score substantially lower (e.g., more than 1.5 standard deviations lower) than the mean normative score.

The third criterion refers to associated difficulties in academic achievement (mathematics), fine-motor skills, and social interaction. Mathematics has historically been a key factor for a diagnosis of NLD, but caution is necessary due to the variety of aspects involved in mathematical learning. Forrest (2004) made the point (see also Spreen, 2011) that the difficulties in mathematics observed in children with NLD are not the same as those usually seen in children with some types of mathematical LD—for example, children with NLD do not usually have trouble recalling arithmetic facts. In fact, neuroimaging research has shown that arithmetic fact retrieval is associated with verbal processes (Grabner et al., 2009), aligning with Geary's (2004) "verbal" subtype of mathematics LD. On the contrary, children with NLD are likely to make visuospatial errors in written calculations (e.g., confusing columns, carrying/borrowing errors) and when writing mirrored numbers (see Osmon, Smerz, Braun, & Plambeck, 2006).

Mammarella et al. (2010a; see also Venneri et al., 2003) showed that arithmetic difficulties are typically associated with NLD, but also argued that this happens only to the extent to which visuospatial processes are involved. This would explain why the pattern of mathematics challenges seen in children with NLD may emerge more clearly from a qualitative analysis than from the overall scores in a standardized test, in which children may partly compensate with their intact verbal skills. Hence, our recommendation is that the diagnosis of NLD should be based on a qualitative analysis of the child's mathematics performance and have specific features, including an average or above-average performance in some verbal achievement tasks, particularly in reading decoding, with the consequence of a discrepancy between reading decoding (which is preserved) and mathematics achievement (which is impaired). Furthermore, mathematics achievement should be cautiously considered in first and second graders. In fact, Drummond et al. (2005) pointed out that this criterion cannot strictly be applied if the NLD label is used prior to third grade, before a stable measure of academic achievement is feasible.

As anticipated in the third criterion, it must be added that the diagnosis is further supported by the presence of other associated symptoms frequently present in the child with NLD. The case of fine-motor impairment seems important as it may also have consequences in school, with reference to handwriting and other skills (e.g., the use of scissors) that may be implied in everyday school activities. In this case, the diagnosis may be also supported by the use of standardized scales that examine fine-motor coordination skills.

Concerning social interaction, it is possible that these difficulties might have more adaptive consequences during adolescence. As Grodzinsky et al. (2010) suggested, social interaction impairments should manifest both at home and school, and should be measured by clinical interview and observation. As these aspects are not easy to assess using psychological tests, we suggest administering behavior rating scales and clinical interviews to parents and teachers (in Chapter 6, we dedicate a paragraph to the differential diagnosis concerning this aspect between NLD and ASD).

With regard to exclusion criteria, the NLD profile has historically been used to characterize children with other diagnosed disorders. As Fine et al. (2013) observed, children with a diagnosis of NLD were not

> distinguished from children with neurological conditions such as hydrocephalus, agenesis of the corpus callosum, Turner's, velocardiofacial syndrome, and others, for which Rourke's NLD profile was consistent (e.g., Rourke & Tsatsanis, 1996). Not until the mid-2000s did researchers regularly exclude intellectual disabilities, seizure disorders, acquired brain damage and other medical, neurological and genetic conditions. (p. 216)

We agree with Spreen (2011) that NLD cannot be used as an umbrella term covering various pediatric disorders. In our view, the diagnosis of NLD concerns a developmental disorder best applied in the absence of the above-mentioned diagnoses, similar to the way that children who present with language problems as a result of an extant disorder such as cognitive impairment are not given a diagnosis of specific language disorder. Hence, we strongly suggest excluding children who meet the full criteria for other diagnosed conditions such as ASD or DCD, as well as other primary genetic and/or neurological conditions.

Conclusions

We hope that a definitive set of diagnostic criteria for NLD will find a consensus among researchers and clinicians studying the disorder. To improve knowledge of good practices in this field, a primary aim must be to ensure that all researchers and clinicians are talking about the same category of children when they use the label "nonverbal learning disability." To achieve this, diagnostic criteria should be defined as clearly as possible. We lay no claim to our criteria being certain and/or final; instead, they should be seen as an attempt to start bringing order to 30 years of wide-ranging research.

It is worth noting that Spreen (2011) argued that children with NLD are not prototypical examples of cases with LD because many of their impairments are not academic in the usual sense, and not as *specific* as the definition of LD suggests. Children with LD are characterized by a marked discrepancy between their general intellectual ability and their academic achievements in reading, writing, or calculation. The analysis of the literature has demonstrated, on the other hand, that few symptoms for diagnosing NLD concern academic achievement (e.g., mathematical skills, handwriting), but these children may have other difficulties that need to be considered (see Cornoldi et al., 2003) in academic areas such as drawing, geography, and so on, as a consequence of their weaknesses in visuospatial processing. Unlike children with other forms of LD, children with NLD may have academic weaknesses, but not always dramatically poor school results. The academic difficulties of children with NLD may also correlate with emotional and social problems, which are typically considered an exclusion criterion for the diagnosis of LD.

As the focus on LD may be misleading, the label "nonverbal disability" is similarly confusing. A more aptly descriptive term may be "specific nonverbal disorder" or "specific visuospatial disorder," so that the label reveals the nature, rather than the absence, of the problem. Given the now widespread use of the term NLD, however, and in the absence of any consensus, the term NLD seems to remain as the most readily comprehensible for the time being. If the criteria for a diagnosis of NLD are clear and broadly shared, this will benefit research and practice, making both less open to misinterpretation. In particular, researchers could examine many aspects that are still unclear in more detail and in well-defined groups.

We are certain that an appropriate diagnosis of NLD can be helpful to researchers and clinicians, and particularly for the children involved and their families, since it draws attention to children who have several problems, but who do not fit into other diagnostic categories. Within this perspective, in the present chapter, we tried to propose possible criteria for its diagnosis in order to improve research and practice in this field. We welcome further discussion and evidence as our understanding of these children progresses.

CHAPTER SIX

Differential Diagnosis and Assessment of Children with NLD

The assessment of a child with NLD follows the same phases of the diagnostic process typical of other developmental disorders. Utilizing best practice for assessment necessitates proper training, use of instruments with the most recent normative standardization data, attention to rapport, and use of multiple informants and sources that test alternate hypotheses. As with any good diagnosis, there should be present a consistency of the data rather than a single isolated score, reporter, or observation form confirmation. The assessment process should include the following steps: parent interview, generation of alternative hypotheses, hypothesis testing (assessment and information discovery via interviews, record review, and direct observation), formulation of diagnosis, and feedback to the parents if the diagnosis is within a clinical rather than a research framework. In this chapter, we discuss important information to gather during the interview, possible alternative hypotheses to consider, and instruments that may be helpful in direct (testing) and informant-based (rating scale) assessment of functioning.

Background Interview

A very thorough interview is the first step in the assessment process, and it is during this construction of a clear developmental history when an alternate hypothesis should initially be generated. Both parents should be present, if possible, to hear multiple perspectives; get a picture of the family dynamics; and to understand the psychological, educational, and social heritable characteristics of the child to be assessed. Be sure that parents bring school report cards and/or teacher reports, copies of any current or past support provided from other professionals such as occupational therapists and speech and language therapists, as well as any baby books or records that will help them to recall their child's developmental history. Samples of work production, including homework or schoolwork, can also be quite helpful along with information on lengths of time to produce written work relative to classmates.

Medical and Developmental History

Medical and developmental history is critical to determining how organic and environmental events might contribute to symptoms. Complete information about childbirth, including medications and substances taken during pregnancy, are important to document as many symptoms related to NLD can occur with fetal alcohol syndrome (Kodituwakku, 2007) and antiepileptic medications, for example (Bolton et al., 2011). Similarly, information about birth weight, fetal maturity, anoxia, and possible hemorrhagic events are also critical to know. Developmentally, one will want to understand how and when language emerged as well as fine-motor milestones. The developmental history should include probes that will serve to rule in or out a diagnosis of ASD (see "Differential Diagnosis," below) as well as medical conditions such as spina bifida, velocardiofacial syndrome, and seizures. Information about past and current sleep hygiene, eating habits, and any information regarding concussion with loss of consciousness, medications, and sensory functioning including data from the most recent hearing and vision exams should be taken because these can influence current functioning, including the direct assessment phase of the process. Within the developmental history for NLD, one might expect to hear that language emerged well and timely.

Family History

When gathering information about family history, it is important to ask about the educational, psychological, and social functioning of biological relatives. Documenting the presence or absence of LD, ASD, ADHD, and psychological health issues can help in generating and ruling out the likelihood of alternative hypotheses. The family configuration and psychosocial stressors that might influence behaviors past and present are also important to record.

Academic and Psychosocial Functioning

For children with NLD, symptoms consistent with the disorder should be observed between the ages of 3 and 5 years. These include poor inclination to draw or to perform fine-motor activities (e.g., completing puzzles, playing with constructional toys such as LEGOs), or in acquiring complex motor skills (e.g., riding a tricycle or bicycle). A difficulty in discriminating or estimating quantity such as comparison of magnitude may be present. During primary school, the symptoms are likely to emerge more clearly, with demonstration of both strengths and weaknesses associated with NLD. Strengths should be observed in verbal activities (e.g., reading decoding and recitation of mathematics facts) and difficulties seen in handwriting, conceptual mathematics, geometry, and mathematics-based science. During latency and adolescence socialization problems could also be reported by parents, with few interactions with other children of the same age and preferred interactions with adults or younger children.

The interview is critical to understanding a child within his or her ecological contexts at home and school. Notably, the process we recommend is generally considered best practice and is reviewed in several books on neuropsychological assessment, including *Neuropsychological Evaluation of the Child* (Baron, 2004) and *Neuropsychological Assessment* (Lezak, 1976). Following the interview, selection of instruments to test hypotheses can begin. For our discussion of the assessment procedures to establish differential diagnoses, we refer to the diagnostic criteria presented in Chapter 5.

Differential Diagnosis

NLD, by definition, presents as a visuospatial deficit along with a constellation of symptoms that could also be found in other disorders. When thinking along dimensional rather than categorical lines, symptoms of many neurodevelopmental disorders are similar, but the relative intensity of specific characteristics may inform the categorical DSM (American Psychiatric Association, 2013) or ICD (World Health Organization, 1992) designation. In NLD, we expect a core problem in visuospatial functioning with a variety of additional symptoms that could be shared with other disorders, but may be less intense than required for a diagnosis of those disorders. For example, a child with NLD may have some social challenges similar to children with ASD, but children with NLD do not meet criteria for a diagnosis on the autism spectrum.

Autism Spectrum Disorder

NLD and ASD can be differentiated by the absence in children with NLD of restrictive/repetitive patterns of behaviors, interests, or activities that are commonly intense in children with ASD. Among the autism spectrum, one of the profiles often confused with NLD is AS (DSM-IV-TR; American Psychiatric Association, 2000) or HFA (DSM-5; American Psychiatric Association, 2013). Asperger syndrome/high-functioning autism (AS/HFA) may be diagnosed when individuals demonstrate the impaired social reciprocity and atypical interests and activities seen in autism, but show no delays in their early language development. Thus, structural language is, at least superficially, a strength both in AS/HFA (Landa, Klin, & Volkmar, 2000) and NLD. It has been suggested that individuals with AS/HFA and NLD also share pragmatic difficulties, including unusual prosody, verbose speech, difficulties interpreting jokes and figurative language in conversation, and lack of response to nonverbal social cues (Klin, Volkmar, Sparrow, Cicchetti, & Rourke, 1995; Ryburn, Anderson, & Wales, 2009; Semrud-Clikeman & Glass, 2008), but these symptoms are more specific and more severe in the case of AS/HFA. Furthermore, the absence of restrictive patterns of interests in children with NLD has been the basis of differential diagnoses between NLD and autism (Semrud-Clikeman, Walkowiak, Wilkinson, & Christopher, 2010a). Although some children with AS/HFA may show difficulty with visuospatial reasoning, this feature is not consistent among children with autism. Thus, children with NLD are generally expected to perform more poorly than those with AS/HFA in visuospatial intelligence and visuoconstructive abilities (Semrud-Clickeman et al., 2010a).

Social (Pragmatic) Communication Disorder

This disorder, also included in DSM-5, is characterized by difficulties in the social use of verbal and nonverbal communication. Children with social (pragmatic) communication disorder (SCD) show severe difficulties in using communication for social purposes (e.g., difficulties with changing communication according to the context, following rules of conversation, making inferences and understanding ambiguous meanings of language, and using nonverbal body and face communicative signs). These difficulties may also be present in NLD but in a less severe way and are not the specific element characterizing the child's difficulties, as they imply other problems. In fact, in contrast to children with SCD, children with NLD might show problems in making inferences (Worling et al., 1999), but specifically reveal problems in processing visuospatial information and show lower visuospatial than verbal intelligence (Mammarella & Cornoldi, 2014) in addition to pragmatic language problems.

Developmental Coordination Disorder

Children with DCD have coordinated motor skills that are substantially below what is expected for children of the same chronological age (American Psychiatric Association, 2013; World Health Organization, 1992). Difficulties are characterized by clumsiness and slowness, and inaccuracy in performing motor skills such as catching objects, riding a bike, or participating in sports. Some of these symptoms may be found in children with NLD in which impairments in fine-motor skills and handwriting are often present. However, in children with DCD many NLD symptoms—and in particular difficulties in processing visuospatial information—are not always present and are not specific (see Alloway & Archibald, 2008).

Specific Learning Disorders

DSM-5 considers as a unique category children with specific learning disorders covering impairment in reading, written expression, and mathematics. The comorbidity between NLD and specific learning disorders may be high and sometimes a diagnosis of LD may be attributed to a case of NLD. In particular, we expect a great presence of mathematics disability in children with NLD. However, the main difference, with respect to many cases of mathematics LD, is related to the nature of the impairment. Geary (2004) suggests that there are three subtypes of mathematics disability related to deficits in either (1) procedural processing, (2) semantic deficits, and (3) visuospatial processing. Children with NLD are likely to align with Geary's third subtype, visuospatial, showing problems in spatial representation, placement of values along a number line, aligning columns, working with decimals, and omission or rotation of numbers (Mazzocco & Myers, 2003). In contrast, children with a specific mathematics disability who do not have NLD are likely to have difficulty with rote mathematics facts (semantic subtype) or in sequencing and in the performance of multistep execution in problem solving (procedural subtype). Thus some, but not all, children with a specific LD in mathematics may also meet criteria for NLD.

Attention-Deficit/Hyperactivity Disorder

NLD may share some similarities with ADHD, in particular for inattentive symptoms referred to as difficulties in organizing tasks and activities. Although children with NLD may fail in visual sustained attention tasks, they often perform well on concomitant verbal tasks. In contrast, children with ADHD show *global* difficulties in maintaining attention to both verbal and visual stimuli. In addition, possible difficulties in visuospatial tasks can be explained by inattentive symptoms in children with ADHD. As mentioned for other disorders, lower visuospatial than verbal intelligence has not been documented within the

ADHD population, nor have poor fine-motor skills, difficulties in perceiving organized forms, and in reproducing simple drawings by copy or memory (Semrud-Clickeman et al., 2010a).

In sum, the above are some examples of important rule-out diagnoses when NLD is a possible hypothesis. In assessment, it is important to use a variety of instruments that can help differentiate the disorders because, behaviorally, children with each of these developmental problems can behave similarly. However, differing neurological processes may underlie the behaviors, thus requiring different interventional programs.

Assessment Instruments

Questionnaires

During the assessment phase it may be useful to use questionnaires and self-report scales to directly collect information from parents, teachers, and the children as well, regarding behaviors at home and school. Questionnaires and checklists are rapid and low-cost tools for collecting information from the child or from those who are familiar with the child, particularly teachers when the child cannot be directly interviewed. Teachers are in contact with children for long periods of time, have a prolonged experience, and have the possibility of comparing behaviors, skills, and motivations of a single child with the whole class. For this reason, their evaluation of the child could offer a significant contribution to the assessment and, despite its limitations, is typically more reliable than that offered by parents (DuPaul et al., 2016). It is important to note that questionnaires are not diagnostic tools, but may be useful to integrate the information derived from the interview with parents and the results obtained from standardized tests.

Broad-spectrum questionnaires that assess the overall psychosocial functioning of children are important for screening out many possible problems—such as anxiety, depression, and attentional issues—when assessing any child for neurodevelopmental disorders. However, there is only one rating scale that is designed specifically to assess symptoms of visuospatial deficits: The Shortened Visuo-Spatial (SVS) Questionnaire (Cornoldi et al., 2003) is a checklist for teachers that was developed in Italy and is translated into other languages. There is also a recent version involving self-report for children (Ferrara & Mammarella, 2013) that captures the awareness of the child about his or her difficulties.

SVS Questionnaire for Teachers

The SVS Questionnaire (Cornoldi et al., 2003) is a checklist for teachers devoted to collecting information about the presence of NLD symptoms within the classroom environment. The questionnaire includes 18 items and uses a 4-point Likert scale (see Appendix 6.1). Ten items concern some of the deficits that, according to previous studies, represent the critical features of NLD. In particular, items include the child's use of the available space on paper while drawing; visuomotor coordination; comprehension of visuospatial relations from verbal description; coordination of complex movements; handling of the spatial components of calculation; orientation to space, drawing, visuospatial learning, and skills in observing the surrounding environment; and ability to deal with novel objects. These items are used to obtain a visuospatial score. The questionnaire also includes two items to evaluate aspects typically associated with NLD, but these scores are not included in the total score. They concern handling of interpersonal skills (item 9) and mathematical learning (item 11). Two items (items 13 and 14) collect preliminary information evaluating the presence of comorbidity with ADHD (see Sandson, Bachna, & Morin, 2000). Finally, four more items are included as a control. They collect information on a child's verbal abilities (items 1 and 10), the teacher's estimate of the child's overall cognitive potential (item 17), and sociocultural level in general (item 18). Normative data based on 4,026 children from third to fifth grade (Cornoldi et al., 2003) and on 1,072 children from sixth to eighth grade (Pedroni, Molin, & Cornoldi, 2007) have been collected (see Table 6.1). A study developed in Italy and Scotland comparing children with different diagnoses has documented the discriminative power of the SVS.

In 2013, Ferrara and Mammarella devised a version of the SVS Questionnaire for self-report of children. The questionnaire includes 15 items derived from the original teacher version (Cornoldi et al., 2003), and most of the items evaluate the child's

TABLE 6.1. Cutoff Scores of the SVS Questionnaire for Children (SVS-C) and for Teachers (SVS-T) Evaluating Visuospatial Skills, According to Grades 3, 4, and 5

Visuospatial score	Third grade	Fourth grade	Fifth grade
SVS-C	< 14	< 15	< 16
SVS-T	< 25	< 25	< 25

awareness about his or her visuospatial difficulties. In particular, six items concern visuospatial and motor skills (e.g., visuomotor coordination, coordination of complex movements, orientation to space, and ability to recall visuospatial information), three items collect information on the child's verbal abilities, two items collect preliminary information evaluating the presence of comorbidity with ADHD, three items collect information about academic achievement, and one item concerns the child's social abilities. Children are asked to evaluate their characteristics on a 4-point scale (see Appendix 6.1); normative data, based on the responses of 886 children from third to fifth grade, have been collected (Ferrara & Mammarella, 2013). In Table 6.1 we report the cutoff scores proposed for the two questionnaires.

Omnibus Rating Scales

Broad rating scales explore the presence of symptoms that can be the focus of clinical concern. There are several scales that gather data from parents, teachers, and children themselves. Many, like the Child Behavior Checklist (CBCL) and the Teacher Report Form (Achenbach, 1991), include scales for psychosocial adjustment and behaviors at home and school. The CBCL has been translated into many languages and consists of a number of statements about the child's behavior. The school-age version contains 120 questions and responses are given on a 3-point Likert scale. The parent (or another caregiver who knows the child well) is asked to answer to a series of items describing children's characteristics. There is also a child-report form: the Youth Self-Report. These scales are used as a diagnostic tool for a variety of behavioral and emotional problems such as ADHD, conduct disorder, childhood depression, separation anxiety, childhood phobia, social phobia, and so on. Scores for internalizing and externalizing problems can be also obtained.

Another broad rating scale, the BASC-2 (Reynolds & Kamphaus, 2004), includes many of the same scales as the Achenbach (1991) rating forms, but also includes questions regarding social adjustment, leadership, and social communication. There are parent-, teacher-, and child-report forms that include both true/false and 3-point Likert questions. As of the writing of this book, the third edition of the BASC is anticipated for release.

Questionnaires for Assessing Clinical Depression and Anxiety

Although empirical evidence does not clearly support clinical depression and anxiety as specifically associated with NLD above any other learning challenge, children who struggle with school and social life are at risk for secondary symptoms related to mood (Rourke & Fuerst, 1992). There are some rating scales designed to probe symptoms of anxiety or depression in children. The Children's Depression Inventory 2 (CDI-2; Kovacs, 2010) is a comprehensive multirater assessment of depressive symptoms in youth ages 7–17 years that can be used in both educational and clinical settings to evaluate depressive symptoms in children and adolescents. It consists of 28 items and yields a total score, which can be divided into two scale scores (i.e., emotional problems and functional problems). Versions for parents, teachers, and children are available. This behavior rating scale should be used in particular with adolescents with NLD for whom the clinician hypothesizes serious difficulties in emotional and social abilities.

The Revised Children's Manifest Anxiety Scale (RCMAS-2; Reynolds & Richmond, 2008) and the Multidimensional Anxiety Scale for Children, Second Edition (MASC-2; March, 2012) are specific child self-report rating scales for identifying children at risk for symptoms of anxiety within the clinical level of concern. These scales rely on child report; results should be carefully interpreted within the context of other collected data including child, parent, and teacher interviews, as well as formal assessment and observations within the school environment. Anxiety can be a significant symptom warranting clinical attention as it can for any child with learning and neurodevelopmental challenges.

Autism Symptom Rating Scales and Interviews

Because it is so important to rule out ASD when assessing children suspected of having NLD, autism measures should be included in the battery. The Social Communication Questionnaire (Rutter, LeCouteur, & Lord, 2003) is a checklist that can be used to screen for symptoms of ASD that might warrant a closer look. This instrument has been shown to discriminate between ASD and non-ASD populations and is considered to be useful as a first-level screener for ASD in school-age children (Chandler et al., 2007). The measure has been translated into several languages, including Chinese (Gau et al., 2011) and German (Bölte, Holtmann, & Poustka, 2008). Other autism screening scales include the Autism Spectrum Rating Scale (ASRS; Goldstein & Naglieri, 2010), the Gilliam Autism Rating Scale, Third Edition (GARS-3; Gilliam, 2013), the Childhood Autism Rating Scale, Second Edition (CARS-2; Schopler, Van Bourgondien, Wellman, & Love, 2010), and the Krug's Asperger Disorder Index (KADI; Krug & Arick, 2003), which all have multiple language translations. If autism is suspected, further evaluation to rule out this diagnosis can be accomplished with the Autism Diagnostic Interview, Revised (ADI-R; LeCouteur, Lord, & Rutter, 2003) and the Autism Diagnostic Observation Schedule, Second Edition (ADOS-2; Rutter, DiLavore, Rsi, Gotham, & Bishop, 2012). If the child meets criteria for autism, then a diagnosis of NLD should not be given, even though some symptoms consistent with NLD may be present. These symptoms might be a focus of intervention, but primary treatment should be with empirically based interventions for children with ASD.

Questionnaires for Assessing Motor Coordination

Questionnaires examining the presence of motor-coordination problems may be useful and may integrate the interviews with parents and other people who know the child. There are many questionnaires examining this point that have been adapted and standardized in different countries, including Italy. Some examples include the Movement Assessment Battery for Children—2 (Movement ABC-2; Henderson, Sugden, & Barnett, 2007), the Motor Observation Questionnaire for Teachers (MOQ-T;

Schoemaker, 2008) and the Developmental Coordination Disorder Questionnaire 2007 for parents (DCDQ'07; Wilson, Kaplan, Crawford, & Roberts, 2007).

Standardized Tests

Assessment of Intelligence (Criterion A)

As mentioned in Chapter 5, a persistent deficit in one or more measures of nonverbal intelligence or reasoning (e.g., perceptual reasoning, visuospatial intelligence) in the presence of an average or above-average verbal intelligence can be considered a primary indicator of NLD. Therefore, for children with NLD the assessment of intelligence should be based on a multicomponent scale of intelligence, capable of detecting good verbal and poor visuospatial intellectual skills. To this purpose, in the case of NLD (and not only NLD), the most used tool is represented by the Wechsler scales. According to our criteria, a persistent deficit in one or more measures of nonverbal intelligence or reasoning in the presence of an average or above-average verbal intelligence should be observed in order to give a diagnosis of NLD.

The different versions of the Wechsler scales (WISC; 1991, 2003, 2014) have been used for the diagnosis of NLD. Traditionally, the reference for the first versions of the WISC concerned the difference between VIQ (high) and PIQ (low) but it was also argued (e.g., Drummond et al., 2005) that only some subtests were crucial. Specifically, in the case of NLD, only a subset of verbal task scores were typically high (i.e., Vocabulary, Similarities, Information) and only a subset of performance task scores were typically low (i.e., Block Design, Object Assembly, Coding).

The WISC-IV battery (Wechsler, 2003) eliminated the Object Assembly subtest, which was one of the subtests with high face validity for discriminating NLD; this was empirically substantiated in one study (Drummond et al., 2005). The fourth edition, however, more clearly defined a visuoperceptual factor. The WISC-IV contains 10 principal subtests and five additional subtests. The age range for the test is between 6 and 16 years, 11 months. The 10 basic subtests yield four indexes: the Verbal Comprehension Index, the Perceptual Reasoning Index, the Working Memory Index, and the Processing Speed Index. In addition,

Full Scale IQ can be computed ranging from 40 to 160 points. A discrepancy between the Verbal Comprehension and Perceptual Reasoning indexes has been historically used as one of the main characteristics of children with NLD (Fine et al., 2013). However, the high incidence of a discrepancy between then VIQ and PIQ in the standardization sample has raised doubts about the utility of this measure, when the difference is below one standard deviation. Moreover, the four indexes indicated in the WISC-IV manual (Wechsler, 1974) do not necessarily propose the best description of the structure of intelligence as measured by the WISC-IV (Keith, Fine, Taub, Reynolds, & Kranzler, 2006). Particularly, within the Perceptual Reasoning Index, a more pure specific visuospatial component may be distinguished from a subfactor best recognized as fluid reasoning. In principle, NLD difficulties should be more associated with the specific than with the central component. Notably, the most recent version of the WISC (WISC-V; Wechsler, 2014), the fifth edition, attempts to address this problem.

The WISC-V takes into account the critical appraisal of previous versions and provides separate factor indexes for fluid reasoning and visuospatial skills, both of which are nonverbal in nature. Based on a general qualitative review of the subtests, two new subtests look as though they may well discriminate children with NLD. The Figure Weights subtest requires the child to estimate and compare the equivalence of visual symbols based on quantity and relative value. The more difficult items require symbolic transformation, with visual WM demands. Based on the work of Mammarella and Cornoldi (2014), deficits in VSWM may be among the most predictive skills in NLD. Visual Puzzles, the second new nonverbal task, requires the synthesis of parts to whole construction including mental rotation, which also requires VSWM. The WISC-V primary indexes comprise two subtests each: The Fluid Reasoning Index includes the Figure Weights and Matrix Reasoning subtests, while the Visual Spatial Index comprises Block Design and Visual Puzzles. The WISC-V also yields a broad Nonverbal Ancillary Index, which is composed of Block Design, Visual Puzzles, Matrix Reasoning, Figure Weights, Picture Span, and Coding. Picture Span is a supplemental subtest that tests short-term memory for object pictures that are easily mediated verbally. Thus, a verbal strategy could be used to achieve good scores, and so this test may be an interesting foil to the Corsi Block-Tapping Task (see "Visuospatial Short-Term Memory and WM") or other visuospatial memory tasks (e.g., dot location from the Test of Memory and Learning [TOMAL-2]; Reynolds & Voress, 2007; finger windows from the Wide Range of Memory and Learning–Revised [WRAML-2]; Sheslow & Adams, 2003) but may also describe the presence of good verbal strategies. Although no empirical data are available yet for the NLD population, the new WISC-V may improve our ability to observe deficits in visuospatial functioning that could aid in diagnosis.

Other measures of intelligence offer separate scores for verbal and visuospatial reasoning. For example, the Kaufman Brief Intelligence Test, Second Edition (KBIT-2; Kaufman & Kaufman, 2004) is a brief, individually administered measure of verbal and nonverbal intelligence. Three different scores can be obtained: verbal, nonverbal, and an overall IQ based on six subtests. The verbal subtests measure crystallized ability and the nonverbal subtests measure fluid reasoning. Also, the classical Primary Mental Abilities Test (PMA; Thurstone & Thurstone, 1963), explicitly based on the assumption of different forms of intelligence, can be useful and is still used in some countries. It appears as a valid instrument for a first large screening of a group of children with NLD, as it is a paper-and-pencil test that can be administered simultaneously. The primary mental abilities assessed by the different versions of PMA can vary, but in Thurstone and Thurstone's model the main abilities are verbal comprehension, word fluency, number facility, spatial visualization, associative memory, perceptual speed, and reasoning. Different subtests according to the child's age were developed for each ability. These abilities partly reflect those individuated in the Cattell–Horn–Carroll (CHC) model (McGrew, 2009); tests referring to the CHC model and offering separate measures of verbal and spatial intelligence can be used for diagnosis of NLD. Finally, the Differential Ability Scales, Second Edition (Elliot, 2006) provide Verbal, Spatial, and Nonverbal Reasoning Indexes that can be used to observe specific problems in visual versus verbal functioning; the Stanford–Binet, Fifth Edition (Roid, 2003) offers separate Verbal and Nonverbal Indexes.

Assessment of Visuospatial Processing (Criterion B)

According to the second criterion suggested by us (see Chapter 5) substantial difficulties in processing visuospatial information should be observed in order to give a diagnosis of NLD, as manifested by at least two of the following weaknesses:

- Difficulties in perceiving organized forms.
- Visuoconstructive impairments including difficulties in drawing, reproducing simple drawings by copy or memory, and reconstructing objects.
- Difficulties in temporarily remembering and manipulating visuospatial information.

In the following paragraphs, a suggestion of possible instruments for measuring these aspects is proposed.

VISUAL PERCEPTION

For the assessment of visuoperceptual abilities, several subtests of the Motor-Free Visual Perception Test (MVPT-3; Colarusso & Hammill, 2003) can be employed for the diagnosis of children with NLD. It is a widely used, standardized test and unlike other visual perception tasks, the MVPT-3 also assesses visual perception independent from motor ability. It was originally developed, based on other previous tasks, for use with children (Colarusso & Hammill, 1972), but the most recent version of the measure can be administered to individuals from 4 to 70 years old. Five areas are assessed: spatial relationship, figure–ground discrimination, visual discrimination, visual closure, and visual memory. However, evidence on this test in association with NLD is scarce, and, with reference to the crucial difficulty in gestalt perception, some subtests could be more critical; also, there are other tasks that could be used as suggested by Mammarella and Pazzaglia (2010).

In the Developmental Test of Visual–Motor Integration (VMI; Beery, Buktenica, & Beery, 2010), a subtest of visual perception is included in which children find the exact figure matched to the target among a series of distractors. It is important to note that the standardization of the visual perception subtest requires that it immediately follows the figure-drawing task. Finally, the Judgment of Line Orientation (JLO; Benton et al., 1994) is a measure of spatial perception without a motor component. The child is asked to look at an array of lines, then is shown two lines, and finally is asked to match the two lines to the array. The NEPSY-II (Korkman, Kirk, & Kemp, 2007) has a similar subtest called Arrows, which is a JLO-like task suitable for children between the ages of 5 and 16. Recently, it has also been argued that basic aspects of vision could be impaired in NLD—for example, Cornetti (2015) offered support to the hypothesis that children with NLD may have an impaired stereoscopic vision. These results suggest that the assessment of visual sensory processes could be taken into consideration in a complete evaluation of children with NLD.

VISUOCONSTRUCTIVE SKILLS

Several measures of visuoconstructive skills have been developed. For the diagnosis of NLD a traditional measure was the Object Assembly subtest present in the first versions of the WISC (Drummond et al., 2005). As previously mentioned, the test is no longer available to clinicians who have the most recent versions of the WISC. At the moment, the most widely used tools for the assessment of visuoconstructive skills are probably the VMI and the Rey Complex Figure and Recognition Trial (Meyers & Meyers, 1995), or some other variation of the Rey Complex Figure Test (Rey, 1941; Osterrieth, 1944; see below). The VMI is inspired by previous tests and in particular by the Bender Visual Motor Gestalt Test developed by Bender (1946) under the inspiration of Gestalt psychology (e.g., Koffka, 2013). The Bender test examines the ability of children to perceive and copy simple figures offering a strong gestalt organization. The test had success and was adapted and subjected to several scoring methods (see, e.g., Koppitz, 1975) and is still largely used in many countries.

In the VMI, the child is similarly asked to copy geometric figures having an overall cohesive configuration. Drawings are presented in order of increasing difficulty and are described with reference to the typical age when they are correctly copied. Figure 6.1 offers an example of a cube, the interior of an

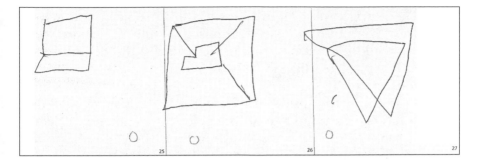

FIGURE 6.1. Examples of VMI stimuli copied by a child with NLD (age 10 years, 7 months).

asymmetrical box, and two double-line intersecting triangles as they were copied by a child with NLD.

Another popular test that is influenced by Gestalt psychology and seems particularly adequate for the diagnosis of NLD was devised by Rey (1941) and later enriched by Osterrieth (1944), and is usually named the Rey Complex Figure Test or some variation of that name. Many scoring procedures have been developed for the test. In the basic version, a complex abstract geometric figure, with an organized but meaningless structure, must be copied and recalled after a few minutes. As the figure includes simple geometric elements, no particular drawing skills are necessary. However, the complexity and strong organization of the elements require that the examinee perceives the structure of the figure and takes into account all the included elements with their patterns and spatial relationships. The main score in the test is represented by the accuracy of the drawing: for each of the 18 elements of the figure the clinician must assess if the element is correctly reproduced and correctly located. Standardized scores for children have been developed for the Meyers and Meyers (1996) scoring system, which also includes normative data for redrawing the figure after 20 minutes. Additionally, there is a motor-free recognition condition that requires the examinee to select the geometric elements and organizing features of the figure from a field of nontarget elements. This condition is helpful for ruling out visual perception problems apart from motor planning and drawing.

The Rey Complex Figure Test has been subjected to many analyses. Rey (1941) himself proposed a simpler version for younger children, but it seems less crucial for the diagnosis of NLD. Other authors have proposed parallel versions or scoring methods of the figure (e.g., Lezak, 1976). However, the main development of the test is associated with the scoring system, which has been refined and accounts for the qualitative aspects of the subject's reproduction, starting from the early phases of the figure construction. From the perspective of the diagnosis of NLD, the early differentiation proposed by Osterrieth (1944) seems crucial, as it distinguishes different pathways by which the subject progressively produces the copy or the reproduction of the figure. A high-level approach to the figure is to recognize the large rectangle as a major organizational feature, and to anchor smaller elements within it. Typically, individuals with NLD do not use these pathways (as shown in the example in Figure 6.2) and this is well visible in the protocol if they are asked to change colors during the drawing. More recently, it has been suggested (Lopez, Tchanturia, Stahl, & Treasure, 2008) that separately considering the six elements that define the structure might assist in deriving a score that reflects the child's ability to grasp the perceptual coherence of the figure.

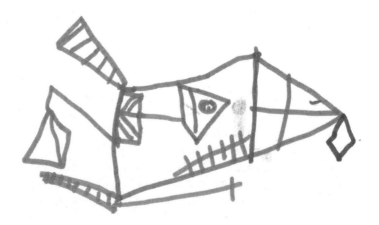

FIGURE 6.2. Example of the Rey Complex Figure copied by a child with NLD (age 10 years, 5 months; average intelligence). The child copied the structure and the details, but did not recognize the large rectangle as a major organizational feature.

There are other tests that provide opportunities to observe visual organization and cohesion. The NEPSY-II includes several subtests ranging from copying designs to motor planning and sequencing. The Design Copy subtest is more structured and less complex than the Rey Complex Figure Test, but it pulls for segmentation more strongly than the simple designs of the VMI. In the Manual Motor Sequences subtest, the child is required to quickly draw a series of lines in a layout. Finally, the route finding subtest of the NEPSY-II requires the child to find a route in a map to reach a specific home target.

VISUOSPATIAL SHORT-TERM MEMORY AND WM

Memory tests that do not involve a visuoconstructive component and require the immediate maintenance or maintenance *plus* processing of visuospatial material are included in this section. The most frequently used test for visuospatial memory is the Corsi Block-Tapping Task, also known as the Spatial Span subtest of the Wechsler Intelligence Scale for Children—Integrated (WISC–Integrated) and the Wechsler Memory Scale (WMS; for adults). The task is inspired by traditional measures used at the beginning of the 20th century for examining visuospatial abilities. In its main current form, the subtest is based on the material and procedure adopted in Brenda Milner's lab in Toronto and used by one of her PhD students, Philip M. Corsi (1972), for his unpublished thesis in order to assess VSSTM span. It can be considered to be the visuospatial analogue of the word and digit spans. The examinee sits opposite the examiner and observes the sequence of blocks on a board (see Figure 6.3) pointed to (tapped) by the examiner. The examinee then indicates the same locations in the same order (forward Corsi span) or in the reverse order (backward Corsi span). The task starts with a small number of blocks and gradually increases up to nine blocks. The presentation stimuli are interrupted when the examinee repeatedly fails with a series of a particular length (see Appendix 6.2 for information about the procedure adopted by Corsi and the series used at the Padua lab, and for indicative normative values). A series of studies (e.g., Mammarella & Cornoldi, 2005b; Basso et al., 2014) has consistently shown that the backward recall is particularly critical in children with NLD.

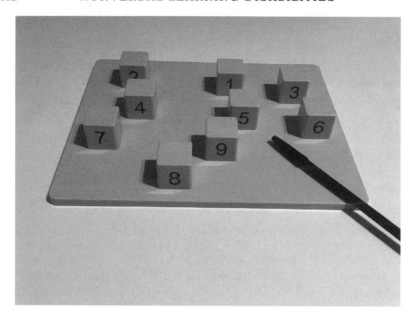

FIGURE 6.3. The Corsi Block-Tapping Task. Numbers on the blocks (not visible to the examinee) can help the examiner in indicating locations with the pointer and in controlling for the accuracy of the response.

The *Padova Visuospatial Battery* was devised at the Learning and Memory Laboratory and associated clinical service for developmental disabilities of the University of Padua, Italy. The battery represents a more systematic tool for the examination of VSWM—the initial focus of research studies in the lab. It involves a further selection and refinement of tasks developed in the lab and already presented in preceding publications (see, in particular, Cornoldi et al., 1997; Cornoldi & Vecchi, 2003) or derived from the literature and adapted to specific research aims.

The battery includes tasks assessing reconstruction of figures (see example in Figure 6.4), comprehension of spatial sentences and visual reproduction of their content, memory of objects located in a matrix (see, e.g., Cornoldi et al., 1995), and many other tasks.

In 2008, in correspondence with the publication of the Italian adaptation of the Corsi test, 12 tests assessing three main components of VSWM were included and published in a standardized

Italian test battery (Mammarella, Toso, Pazzaglia, & Cornoldi, 2008b). Nine tests are simple (passive) storage tasks, while three are complex (active) span tasks. The simple storage tasks are computerized and are divided into visual, spatial–sequential, and spatial–simultaneous tasks according to a distinction supported by previous evidence (Pazzaglia & Cornoldi, 1999; Mammarella, Pazzaglia, & Cornoldi, 2008a). The spatial–sequential and spatial–simultaneous tasks involve the same stimuli; only the presentation format (sequential vs. simultaneous) changes. Examples of the tasks used are shown in Figure 6.5.

A change detection–recognition paradigm is used for the simple storage tasks. Examinees have to decide whether a series of figures/locations is the same as or differs from the one previously presented: after a first set of stimuli has been presented, either the same set is presented or a set with just one element changed, followed by a response screen containing two letters: *U* (*uguale* = the same) and *D* (*diverso* = different). Examinees respond by pressing one of two keys on the keyboard. For each test, the correct answer for half the items is "the same," while for the other half it is "different." The tests progress from the second level (involving two stimuli) to the eighth (containing eight stimuli), and include three items at each level.

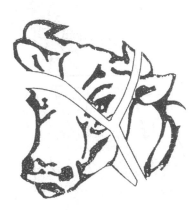

FIGURE 6.4. Example of the puzzle test included in the battery developed by Cornoldi et al. (1997).

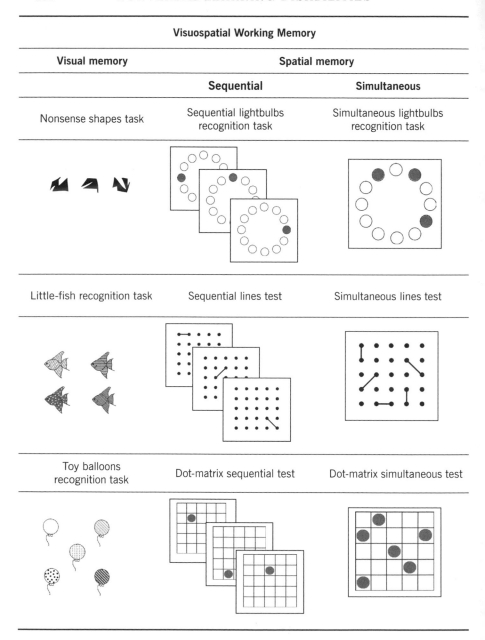

FIGURE 6.5. Examples of tasks included in the VSWM battery (Mammarella et al., 2008b).

In the visual tasks, children are presented with a series of stimuli whose memory cannot be supported by language (meaningless figures, fishes, or balloons with different textures) and asked to decide whether the stimuli of a successively presented series are or are not identical to previously seen stimuli. In the spatial–sequential tests, children are presented with matrices of different shapes in which a series of locations appear one after the other. Then, the child must decide whether the series of locations successively presented is the same or is different. Finally, in the spatial–simultaneous tests, children are presented with patterns of locations appearing at the same time and need to decide whether the new pattern is exactly the same as the one presented just before, or whether a stimulus appeared in a different location.

In the complex span tasks, children have to simultaneously retain and process (1) visual objects (i.e., jigsaw puzzles), (2) spatial–sequential information (i.e., to-be-imagined pathways), and (3) spatial–simultaneous information (i.e., visual patterns to be modified for meeting the recall request). The tests progress from a second level (with two stimuli) to a 10th level (with 10 stimuli), with three items for each level.

The *jigsaw puzzle task* (adapted from Vecchi & Richardson, 2000) consists of drawings developed by Snodgrass and Vanderwart (1980), each of which is broken down into two to 10 numbered pieces, forming a puzzle. Each whole drawing is presented for a few seconds, together with its verbal label, and then removed. The puzzles have to be solved, not by moving the pieces, but by writing down the number corresponding to each piece on a response sheet.

In the *pathway span task* (adapted from Cornoldi et al., 1995), children are required to mentally visualize a pathway followed by a little man moving on a blank matrix. At the end of a series of statements regarding directions given by the experimenter (i.e., forward, backward, left, or right), examinees need to indicate the man's final position in the same matrix. The complexity of the task may vary according to the size of the matrices (from 2×2 to 6×6) and the length of the pathway described.

In the *active version of the visual pattern test* (derived from Della Sala, Gray, Baddeley, & Wilson, 1997), children are presented with filled cells in a matrix that are created by filling in half the cells in the matrix. The matrices increase in size from the smallest (four squares with two cells filled) to the largest (20 squares with 10 cells filled). After the presentation phase, examinees are presented with a blank test matrix on which they have to reproduce the same pattern by filling in the cells but one row *lower down* with respect to the pattern seen in the presentation matrix. For example, if the second cell in the first row of the presentation matrix had been filled, children have to fill in the second cell in the second row in the recall test.

The final scores are obtained from the sum of the three items identified correctly on the most complex levels reached.

Assessment of Motor Coordination, Academic Learning, and Social Abilities (Criterion C)

The third criterion for diagnosing children with NLD proposed in Chapter 5 requires the presence of clinical and/or psychometric indexes of weaknesses in at least one of the following areas:

- Motor coordination.
- Academic achievement in mathematics or other activities involving visuospatial skills in the presence of an average or above-average performance in reading decoding tasks.
- Social interactions.

These three aspects cannot be easily and completely assessed using the standardized procedures available in the clinical services; typically, clinicians also rely on interviews, questionnaires (see "Questionnaires" above), protocol analysis, and clinical observation. However, several standardized measures are available especially in the case of fine-motor abilities.

MOTOR COORDINATION

For the assessment of fine-motor skills, different tasks may be used by clinicians in different countries. However, the tasks included in the NEPSY-II and Movement ABC-2 Test have a more international visibility. In the NEPSY-II (Korkman et al., 2007), several tasks can be used to assess fine-motor skills. In the Fingertip Tapping, the child reproduces simple hand movement sequences, first using the dominant hand and then the nondominant hand. In the Imitating Hand Positions, the child reproduces hand gestures with both the dominant and the nondominant hands. Finally, in the Manual Motor Sequences, the child has to reproduce sequences of hand movements using one or two hands. The Movement ABC-2 Test (Henderson et al., 2007) offers a more general assessment of children's motor coordination and is considered the main tool for the diagnosis of DCD. Many subtests should also be used when diagnosing NLD.

In the Northern American tradition, motor tests largely used in the case of NLD are the Purdue Pegboard, the Grooved Pegboard, and the Finger Tapping Tests. The Purdue Pegboard (Tiffin, 1968) requires the child to place pegs in holes as quickly as possible, first with the dominant hand, then with the nondominant hand, and finally, with both hands together for 30 seconds for each hand. This test is also a good measure of manual dexterity (Reddon, Gill, Gauk, & Maerz, 1988). The Grooved Pegboard (Kløve, 1963) measures complex finger coordination and motor planning. It consists of a board with slotted holes angled in various directions. Each peg has a groove and only fits in one way in each hole. The child first uses the dominant hand and then the nondominant hand to place the pegs as quickly as possible. This test is also a good measure of lateralization impairment (Lezak, Howieson, & Loring, 2004). Finally, the Finger Tapping Test (Reitan & Wolfson, 1985) requires the child to tap a key as quickly as possible, first with the dominant hand and then with the nondominant one.

ACADEMIC ACHIEVEMENT (READING DECODING AND MATHEMATICS)

In order to recognize average reading decoding and poor scores in mathematics achievement, our suggestion is to administer achievement tasks of at least these two measures. Standardized tests typically vary in each country, especially in the case of reading decoding where the assessment must be based on linguistic material calibrated for the specific interested language. With reference to the Anglophone community, WIAT (Breaux, 2009), WRAT (Wilkinson & Robertson, 2006), WJ-Cog III (Woodcock et al., 2001; Woodcock, McGrew, & Mather, 2007), and other test batteries with standardized normative data can be used for assessing both reading and mathematics. The Test of Word Reading Efficiency (TOWRE; Torgesen, Wagner, & Rashotte, 1999) offers timed single-word decoding of both real and pseudowords, requiring only 2 minutes to administer. In any case, as the difficulties presented in mathematics by children with NLD mainly involve the visuospatial aspects of mathematics, consideration of overall mathematics performance should be associated with a more analytical and deep consideration of crucial subtests (e.g., written calculation, geometry) in which errors in the protocols could guide the diagnosis. KeyMath-3 Diagnostic Assessment (Connolly, 2007) has a variety of basic mathematics calculation, applied data analysis (e.g., reading graphs), algebra, and geometry subtests that are given under untimed conditions and may be useful for observing mathematics functioning in specific areas.

SOCIAL INTERACTIONS AND SOCIAL SKILLS

In order to assess associated problems in social interactions of children with a possible diagnosis of NLD, behavior rating scales and clinical interviews (discussed above) represent the most-used tools. However, there are some direct tests of social language and interpersonal problem solving that might prove helpful in directly assessing social reasoning. For example, the Test of Problem Solving (TOPS-3; Bowers, Huisingh, & LoGiudice, 2005) is a test of affective reasoning, which has items for children ages 6–12 years (TOPS-3 Elementary) and ages 12–17 (TOPS-2 Adolescent). The Social Language Development Test (Bowers, Huisingh, & LoGiudice, 2008), also available in child and adolescent versions, assesses language-based social interpretation and reasoning. Both of these tests should be interpreted in light of the overall language development of the child, which should be largely typically developed in children with NLD. The test of affect recognition of NEPSY-II (Korkman et al., 2007) that requires the child to identify basic emotions in the faces of others may also be used. For adolescents and adults, the Social Problem-Solving Inventory—Revised (SPSI-R; D'Zurilla, Nezu, & Maydeu-Olivares, 2002) is a self-report questionnaire that asks examinees to respond to questions about their social problem-solving skills. It yields information about how the examinee makes social decisions; in addition, Spanish normative data are available for the SPSI-R.

Conclusion

The present chapter highlighted the phases of the diagnostic process for children with NLD and offered the most used tests and self-report scales by following the diagnostic criteria presented in Chapter 5. As already mentioned, it is worth noting that self-report scales and questionnaires may be useful tools which give information derived both from teachers and parents, to be integrated with the results obtained in the standardized tests administered to the child. Tests and questionnaires cited in the present chapter should be considered as different alternatives to be used during the assessment phase and their choice should change according to the age of the child or the request of the family. Finally, a crucial aspect in the diagnostic process is represented by the differential diagnosis, in which the clinician develops and considers alternative hypotheses to reach the final diagnosis. In the present chapter, we tried to consider symptoms that could be shared with other disorders (such as ASD, SCD, DCD, LD and ADHD), highlighting the differences with the typical symptoms of children with NLD in order to help clinicians in defining the crucial issues and to guide their diagnostic reasoning.

APPENDIX 6.1

SVS Questionnaire

Shortened Visuo-Spatial Questionnaire for Teachers

Items followed by "VSLD" are used for obtaining the VSLD score (1 = not at all, 2 = sometimes, 3 = most of the time, 4 = completely).

	1	2	3	4
1. Can the child easily memorize material such as names, information, and poems?				
2. Is the child able to make use of the available space when drawing? VSLD				
3. Can the child use tools such as scissors, set square, and ruler, which require independent and coordinated use of both hands? VSLD				
4. Does the child understand spoken commands or texts, which involve spacial relationships? VSLD				
5. Is the child able to execute complex everyday movements (e.g., tying shoelaces)? VSLD				
6. Does the child show a good understanding of spatial relationships in calculation, and can he or she write numbers in a column correctly? VSLD				
7. Does the child have good spatial orientation abilities? VSLD				
8. Is the child good at drawing? VSLD				
9. Can the child easily interact with friends?				
10. Has the child reached a good linguistic learning level for his or her age?				
11. Has the child reached a good mathematics learning level for his or her age?				
12. Is the child competent in learning contexts, which rely on visuospatial skills? VSLD				
13. Is the child distracted easily?				
14. Is the child often restless and/or hyperactive?				
15. Is the child a good observer of the environment in which he or she lives? VSLD				
16. Does the child demonstrate interest in new objects, and can he or she deal with them? VSLD				
17. Does the child show good overall cognitive potential?				
18. Does the child have a poor sociocultural background?				

Shortened Visuo-Spatial Questionnaire for Children

Items followed by "VSLD" are used for obtaining the VSLD score (1 = not at all, 2 = sometimes, 3 = most of the time, 4 = completely).

	1	2	3	4
1. I can easily memorize material such as names, information, and poems.				
2. I like reading.				
3. I am able to use tools such as scissors, set square, and ruler? VSLD				
4. I have good spatial orientation abilities (e.g., in a supermarket I'm able to find the exit easily). VSLD				
5. I am able to execute complex everyday movements (e.g., tying shoelaces). VSLD				
6. I am able to write numbers in a column correctly.				
7. I have good grades in reading.				
8. My exercise books are orderly.				
9. I have good grades in mathematics.				
10. I am easily distracted.				
11. I am often restless and I am not able to stay seated during lessons.				
12. When I am standing in line, I remember who is in front of me and who is behind me. VSLD				
13. When I look at a picture, I am able to recall the details of the image. VSLD				
14. I should be able to reproduce the exact location of the school desks in my class. VSLD				
15. It is easy for me to make friends.				

APPENDIX 6.2

Order of Blocks and Indicative
Normative Values for the Forward and Backward
Corsi Block-Tapping Task

Locations Derived from the Literature in the Forward and Backward Versions

Span levels	Corsi forward			Corsi backward
	Cornoldi & Soresi (1980)	Pagulayan et al. (2006)	Spinnler & Tognoni (1987)	Cornoldi & Soresi (1980)
1		1 9 6 3		
2		57 21 82 37	85 64 18	85 43
3	379 146	436 381 527 614	472 815 958	293 843
4	2973 9438	3249 1765 3571 6849	9315 4987 7532	1946 3925
5	25837 43928	34875 81536 64529 31724	34172 85419 91826	37192 17586
6	184257 283769	568194 416782 259631 792513	236495 981465 231594	685791 238649
7	5293461 7583914	5416973 7193462 9535817 2681495	5947362 6547321 7241836	9468175 8526794
8	25814376 26183954	14728369 59372184 76931548 42139578	18673249 45821793 25817639	

| 9 | | 374192568 752864193 953712648 637425198 | 236748195 894328651 597246318 | |
| 10 | | | 8531974862 2714361589 7894185623 | |

Normative Data According to the Previous Sequences

			Corsi forward		Corsi backward	
Study	Age/grade	N	Mean	SD	Mean	SD
Cornoldi & Soresi (1980)	1st grade	33	4.1	0.7	3.2	0.4
	2nd grade	74	4.3	1.6	3.3	0.8
	3rd grade	41	4.5	1.1	3.8	1.0
	4th grade	46	5.1	0.8	4.6	1.3
	5th grade	83	4.8	0.9	4.6	1.4
Pagulayan et al. (2006)	7 years	26	5.0	0.8		
	8 years	27	5.2	1.0		
	9 years	24	5.5	1.0		
	10 years	24	6.0	1.1		
	11 years	26	6.3	0.9		
	12 years	47	6.3	0.9		
	13 years	32	6.4	0.9		
	14 years	40	6.9	1.1		
	22 years	94	7.1	1.0		
Spinnler & Tognoni (1987)	40–49 years	44	4.8	0.9		
	50–59 years	63	4.5	0.9		
	60–64 years	43	4.4	0.7		
	65–69 years	42	4.2	0.9		
	70–74 years	48	4.1	0.8		
	75–79 years	37	3.7	0.7		
	80–84 years	28	3.7	0.7		
	≤ 85 years	19	3.7	0.8		

CHAPTER SEVEN

Intervention Guidelines and Strategies

Individuals with NLD may present adaptive difficulty in many different life contexts—for example, in school, community, and home. In addition, the challenges faced may change developmentally as the child ages. Therefore, children with NLD need to be supported appropriately with specific interventions and educational strategies according to the developmental and environmental context. In this chapter, we offer an overview of how one might develop intervention procedures that have been mentioned in the literature. It is important to remember that only modest scientific evidence on the efficacy of the proposed procedures has been reported. In fact, the scientific literature on interventions for children with NLD is scarce. The literature primarily includes textbooks written by practitioners or mothers of children with NLD who have in mind specific situations and often refer to children with severe intellectual and emotional problems (i.e., profiles that differ from the most typical NLD profile we have presented in this book). Hence, interventions suggested for children with severe psychosocial and/or intellectual problems, which differ from the diagnosis of NLD presented in this volume, are not considered in the present chapter.

We begin here with a review of the literature followed by the presentation of general guidelines. Next, we present policies that can be adopted in school, family, and community settings in order to support children with NLD. Finally, we suggest approaches that might be taken for psychological intervention. In this chapter, we make reference to the developmental population with NLD, without considering adults with NLD, for which there is no extant research.

Empirical Evidence for NLD Interventions

As mentioned above, empirical evidence on interventions for NLD is scarce. Furthermore, it may also be biased by the fact that treated groups or single cases may not have comparable characteristics; we hope that in the future this gap will be corrected as researchers begin to adopt consistent operational criteria for the diagnosis of NLD. We limit ourselves here to a short overview of empirical evidence on treatment published in the scientific literature. Note that much of the evidence involves the treatment of children who present an NLD profile associated with other neurological problems—for example, with genetic syndromes or who were either generically defined as LD or associated with a mild Asperger profile (e.g., Bonner, Hardy, Willard, & Gururangan, 2009; Swillen et al., 1999). However, in this chapter, we focus on specific NLD profiles not related to other clinical or neurological conditions; therefore, these findings are not considered presently.

In 1991, Foss published a paper titled "Nonverbal Learning Disabilities and Remedial Interventions," summarizing the areas in which interventions for NLD should be focused. Although the paper does not present clear evidence on the effects of intervention, it represents a useful basis for considering the intervention issues. Foss emphasizes that direct instruction in learning strategies are an important aspect of teaching children with NLD. For example, because children with NLD may interpret information related to spatial relationships in a vague or rigid way (p. 133), a multisensory approach that includes training in verbal self-direction may be important. A recommendation that a tutor/teacher and student work together to develop sequences of approach to problems (i.e., developing a meta-analytic system), can help the child develop analytical skills. Foss also addressed production problems in children with NLD, suggesting that poor comprehension may limit written production. Thus, clarifying

semantic relationships through active verbalization and subvo-
calization as a practice by which the child tests his or her own
understanding—for example, "Are there signal words here which
indicate a relationship I should be thinking about?" (p. 136)—
can help lead the child to reflect more on what he or she read.
Written production can increase through automaticity of word
relationships and concepts. Verbal self-instruction is offered as
additionally useful to improve the physical aspects of handwriting, which may be challenging with regard to spacing, speed,
and letter formation. Finally, Foss suggests that it is important
to increase the personal effectiveness of children with NLD
through helping them to master skills.

Taking a similar stance as Foss (1991), Van Luit (2009) examined the influence of explicit verbal instructions on the arithmetic skills of five children with NLD. The study was divided into
three phases: (1) a baseline phase, in which six arithmetic tests
were administered; (2) an intervention phase, in which children
received intervention sessions of 45 minutes twice a week for 10
weeks, divided into 35 minutes of instructions and 10 minutes
of testing; and (3) a posttest phase, in which six parallel arithmetic tests were administered. Verbal instructions followed five
steps. In the first step, the teacher gave a demonstration of the
task and talked aloud. In the second step, the teacher and the
child worked together to perform the same task using verbaliza-
tions. In the third, the teacher and the child worked separately
on the same task, and the child could ask for the support of the
teacher, if necessary. The fourth step had the child finishing the
task alone while verbalizing aloud. Finally, in the fifth step, the
child finished the task guided by self-instruction. Results showed
that all of the children improved in arithmetic skills, although
the target 80% mastery level was obtained only by some children.

There are some studies with children who were not explicitly
defined as having NLD but presented with symptoms typical of
NLD. For example, Litt, Taylor, Klein, and Hack (2005) studied a
group of children with very low birth weight (VLBW group <750
grams), a slightly higher-weight group (750–1,499 grams), and
typically developing controls. All of the children had at least low-
average IQ and no sensory or motor deficits. Children with an
NLD-like profile were most often observed in the VLBW group.
Multiple learning trials and direct instruction were proposed for

teaching such children. Notably, grade retention occurred more frequently in the VLBW group, but the authors suggest that retention may not benefit such children due to the expectation of long-term learning problems in the population.

In recent years, several single-case studies have been conducted with children with NLD; Mammarella, Coltri, Lucangeli, and Cornoldi (2009a) described the efficacy of an intervention on VSWM in an 11-year-old boy with NLD. Both teachers and parents reported that he was impaired in recalling the position of objects, way-finding abilities, and remembering the location of familiar landmarks. Teachers were also worried about his difficulties in arithmetic. The boy showed a VIQ of 94, a PIQ of 75, and a Total IQ of 84. The VSWM battery described in Chapter 6 (Mammarella et al., 2008b)—which involves three tasks assessing the visual component, three the spatial–sequential component, and three the spatial–simultaneous component of WM—was presented before the intervention, after the training, and at the follow-up (after 6 months). The pretraining assessment revealed that the boy specifically failed on spatial–simultaneous tasks. For this reason, training on spatial–simultaneous memory in seven sessions was conducted twice a week for about 50 minutes each session. The intervention was divided into three sessions on recognition of patterns, three on recall of objects presented simultaneously in the test space, and one session for generalizing strategies to everyday life. A consistent sequence of activities was used during each session: explanation of objectives, stimuli presentation, demonstration of the task, questions, feedback, and finally, discussion about the strategies employed to perform the tasks. The results indicated that the training on spatial–simultaneous memory was successful and the improvements were maintained after 6 months. In addition, a near-transfer effect on visual WM tasks was observed immediately after the training. However, at follow-up, the effect of the training remained stable for spatial–simultaneous WM tasks but not for visual WM tasks.

Another single-case study has been reported by Caviola, Toso, and Mammarella (2011) and concerned a 9-year-old girl with NLD. Her intellectual abilities, measured with WISC-III (Wechsler, 1991), were VCI (Verbal Comprehension Index) = 103, POI (Perceptual Organization Index) = 80, FDI (Freedom from Distractibility) = 100, PSI (Processing Speed Index) = 79, and Total

IQ = 90. Detailed psychometric and neuropsychological assessment on VWSM (Mammarella et al., 2008b) revealed deficits in both visual and spatial–sequential WM. The visual WM intervention proposed by Mammarella, Toso, and Caviola (2010b) was given for eight sessions. Results showed a specific improvement of visual tasks, with the benefit of the training maintained after 40 days. The study also observed a transfer effect on geometric achievement, which seemed to be related to the improvements in visual WM.

Finally, Mammarella and Lipparini (2015) describe the case of Matteo, an 11-year-old boy with an NLD profile. He had a Total IQ score of 82 (VCI = 105, POI = 64, FDI = 97, PSI = 82) and his teachers reported difficulties in reading comprehension and study organization. For these reasons, although Matteo was characterized by poor visuospatial abilities, the authors decided to focus the intervention on reading comprehension (10 sessions) and study method (10 sessions). In the first phase of the intervention, he was trained on making inferences, developing reading comprehension strategies, and improving in the integration between written text and figures. In the second phase of the intervention, he was trained to use adequate strategies for studying, organizing materials, and individuating priorities, which were based on Matteo's characteristics. In addition, two sessions were devoted to improve motivation and reduce anxiety prior to taking exams. The results revealed a benefit in both reading comprehension and learning strategies.

Explicitly teaching social skills to children with NLD is an area of intervention that lacks strong empirical support, but which has considerable face validity and some success with other populations such as ASD (Matson, Matson, & Rivit, 2007). The Social Competence Intervention Program (SCIP; Guli, Wilkinson, & Semrud-Clikeman, 2008) is a multisensory manualized 16-session treatment based on creative drama. SCIP aims to improve social functioning by progressing through a process that includes establishing group cohesion, increasing emotional knowledge, learning how to focus attention, recognizing facial and bodily expression, listening to vocal cues, and learning how to put multiple cues together to create understanding (Guli, Semrud-Clikeman, Lerner, & Britton, 2013, p. 40). The intervention has been piloted and tested in children with NLD,

ASD, and ADHD, but without dividing the clinical groups into subtypes. Guli et al. (2013) recently implemented a study using SCIP. Unfortunately, only two children with NLD were in the treatment group, while five were in the control group, thus generalizations on children with NLD are difficult. Postintervention metrics included both rating scales and field observations. Results showed, after a mean approximate number of 24 hours of intervention over the 16 sessions, that acquired social skills including positive interaction and decreased solitary play generalized to the natural school setting. However, it is important to note that the treatment groups were small and mixed, thus it can only be said that children with social deficits can learn and generalize from this type of intervention.

Another drama-based intervention that may indirectly have implications for NLD was implemented over 4 weeks with 90-minute sessions once per week using the Sociodramatic Affective Relational Intervention (SDARI; Lerner, Mikami, & Levine, 2011). SDARI was compared with a commonly used manualized knowledge-based treatment, Skillstreaming (McGinnis & Goldstein, 1997), in children with HFA. No changes in social functioning at home were reported by parents for either treatment group. The authors suggest that this may be the result of a short treatment duration. Children in the SDARI group appeared to make friends within the group more quickly than those in the Skillstreaming group, but although they took more time to evolve, those interactions became more frequent for the Skillstreaming group during unstructured time. It was concluded that, in the HFA population, knowledge-based treatments may work more slowly, but as effectively, as performance-based interventions.

With regard to the response to intervention comparing children with verbal LD and NLD, Yu, Buka, McCormick, Fitzmaurice, and Indurkhya (2006) looked at the long-term downstream behavioral functioning of 8-year-old children who had received parent/family treatment between the ages of 0 and 3 years. The intervention consisted of home visits and implementation of a "child-learning" curriculum given at local centers. The curriculum was intended to improve the cognitive and social skills of the children, all of whom were born low birth weight and premature. NLD and verbal LD were determined by academic area (reading: verbal LD, or math: NLD) and at least one standard deviation lower than Full Scale IQ. Children with verbal LD were found to be twice as likely to have externalizing behaviors (e.g., ADHD and conduct disorders), but NLD was not associated with an increased probability of such behaviors. Internalizing behaviors were not associated with any LD subtype. Early intervention had no influence on the behaviors of any group of children, except that children with verbal LD were *more* likely to be described with internalizing symptoms if they received the treatment. The authors suggest that the training may have made parents more attuned to pathological symptoms while raising the expectation that the intervention should have reduced problem symptoms in their children.

The treatment literature for children with NLD not only is scarce but also has many limitations. These include the absence of robust studies of interventions delivered directly to children with NLD compared with other interventions, clinical groups, or neurotypical children. Although there is some traction for performance-based interventions, it may be that more tradi-tional knowledge-based treatments can work as well, if findings within the autism community can be extended to those with NLD. Future research is needed to better understand how best to intervene socially, academically, and psychologically. Never-theless, there is much speculation and a strong feeling among clinicians about how to proceed in the delivery of interventions for children with NLD.

General Guidelines for Clinical Interventions

The following part of this chapter is based on the material cited above and on experience collected by the authors of the present volume, and presents a set of general guidelines for the clinical intervention with the child with NLD. The following guidelines are general and may also be partly applied to other neurodevel-opmental disorders, but are here considered with reference to the case of NLD. They are inspired by previous guidelines (see Broitman & Davis, 2013; Cornoldi et al., 1997; Davis & Broitman, 2011; Tsatsanis & Rourke, 2003), literature (Foss, 1991; Matte & Bolaski, 1998), and our own experience.

Children with NLD benefit from direct, systematic, and structured instructions, similar to other children with LD. Within this general framework, there are specific principles that may be useful for these children (see Table 7.1). In particular, due to the risks of adaptive impairments, a long-term treatment plan is recommended, supervised by a clinician who can interact systematically and coherently with the different operators who will interact with the child, along the child's course of development. The intervention should take into account the present characteristics of the child and develop a plan that anticipates the most

TABLE 7.1. Guidelines for Treating Children with NLD

1. Define a long-term plan for supporting the child with NLD and identify a clinician assuming the responsibility of its coordination.

2. Base the plan on a precise assessment of the child, the child's adaptive risks, and the context-available resources.

3. Establish priorities, working on one or two things at a time; do not "overload."

4. Use a multimodal approach intervening on the child and on the school, family, and social contexts.

5. Develop awareness in the child of his or her NLD characteristics illustrating both strengths and weaknesses of the NLD profile to build the capacity for self-understanding and self-advocacy.

6. Accept the idea that it will be impossible to eliminate some specific deficits and look for modalities to avoid if they negatively affect the child's general development.

7. Work to prevent the development of secondary symptoms, in particular, related to emotional adjustment.

8. Within a developmental perspective, optimize cognitive skills early on and build on adaptive skills in older children.

9. Help the child to interpret nonverbal communication signs.

10. Increase appropriate self-efficacy and self-effort attributions in order to motivate the child's efforts to change and reduce the risks for learned helplessness.

11. Suggest alternative strategies, and help the child to also think of alternative strategies for coping.

12. Develop metacognitive awareness and verbal strategies for specific situations where the child is in difficulty.

13. Automatize basic procedural knowledge in the areas of difficulty.

14. Avoid an overload of the WM capacity of the child, specifically on visuospatial materials.

15. Divide complex tasks into subobjectives and aid the child to use verbal self-instructions.

serious problems the child is likely to face during development. In fact, due to the large range of problems present in children with NLD, it seems important to establish priorities and support these children with regard to wellness, self-efficacy, and awareness about their own problems. Confer the expectation that overcoming life's difficulties can be accomplished by adopting the appropriate developmental strategies.

The guidelines address both improving the weaknesses present in the child based on a deficit approach, and developing strategies and compensatory mechanisms making the child able to satisfactorily meet life requirements despite retaining some weaknesses. This is coherent with the suggestions advanced by other experts. For example, Telzrow and Bonar (2001; see Table 7.2) summarized the interventions that clinicians, educators, and parents might use with children with NLD, dividing them among remedial interventions designed to train deficient skills directly, use of compensatory instruments such as assistive technology to bypass areas of deficit, and use of specialized methods to teach children foundational strategies to improve skills. Table 7.2 provides some examples of the three types of interventions. Telzrow and Bonar also suggest selecting an approach according to the individual characteristics of the child, including age (e.g., remedial interventions are more effective in younger than older children), severity of deficits, degree of functional impairment, and presence of preserved abilities.

A classical way of treating children with NLD and other specific neuropsychological problems is based on the logic of deficit-centered training. As we have seen, the literature reports a few single-case studies of children treated for a specific problem. Our suggestion is to focus the intervention on visuospatial and visuomotor skills during primary school. As children mature, the intervention should focus on specific skills such as academic areas (mathematics, reading comprehension, and written expression), psychological adjustment, and/or social interaction skills. Regarding these latter skills, assertiveness trainings, interpersonal problem solving, creative drama, and cognitive-behavioral therapy may be useful. An individualized intervention offers the child the experience of feeling understood, appreciated, and discovering strategies to improve social relations and emotional responses.

TABLE 7.2. A Summary of Interventions That Clinicians, Educators, and Parents Might Use with Children with NLD

Remedial interventions	Compensatory instruments	Instructional or therapeutic interventions
Psychomotor and visuoperceptual deficits		
• Direct instruction in functional perceptual skills, such as reading maps and graphs	• Extended time for completion of written tasks • Handwriting aids, such as word processor • Reliance on multiple choice when examining content knowledge • Organizing worksheets with a limited number of clear, well-spaced prompts • Use of oral or written directions and explanations instead of visual maps and schemas	• Early and sustained training and practice in keyboarding skills • Specific training in handwriting accuracy and speed • Specific training in visuospatial abilities
Arithmetic difficulties		
• Direct instruction in computation using verbal mediation to rehearse sequential steps • Instructional/ therapeutic interventions • Verbal rhymes and memory aids to teach mathematics facts • Direct instruction in checking strategies • Rehearsal strategies that rely on verbal mnemonic devices	• Graph paper to assist in column alignment when completing arithmetic problems • Color-coded arithmetic worksheets to cue left–right directionality • Commercially or teacher-prepared chapter summaries and study guides	• Strategy training in specific skill areas, such as written calculation

(continued)

TABLE 7.2. *(continued)*

Remedial interventions	Compensatory instruments	Instructional or therapeutic interventions
	Social interaction deficits	
• Direct instruction in social pragmatic skills, such as making appropriate eye contact, greeting others, and requesting assistance • Teaching strategies for making and keeping friends	• Vocational guidance toward careers that minimize interpersonal skill requirements • Choosing structured, adult-directed, individual, or single-peer social activities over unstructured or large-group events	• Social skills training • Interpersonal rules, social stories, and social scripting • Pragmatic language therapy to address skills related to topic maintenance, verbal self-monitoring, and appropriate social communication

Note. Based on Telzrow and Bonar (2001).

In order to maximize the efficacy of the intervention for the child with NLD, all of the possibilities useful for improving the child's quality of life should be considered. Interventions might include medication to reduce symptoms of anxiety, depression, or inattention. A good plan must necessarily not only be directed to the child but also to the school and family. In the next paragraphs we provide some suggestions for an integrated intervention in which health professionals, teachers, and families are involved.

Health Issues and Medical Interventions

Health and body fitness of children with NLD should be attended to as for any child, but may assume a particular relevance in the case of NLD. In fact, due to psychomotor problems and shyness, children with NLD may be less involved in physical activity than their peers. Concerning the use of drugs, it is worth noting that, at the moment, available medications do not directly treat the basic neurocognitive features of children with NLD. However, just as with other neurodevelopmental disorders, medications may be useful in treating associated symptoms. Severe mental problems for NLD have not been verified in the literature, nor observed in our experience, but in some cases a psychiatric intervention including drug prescription might be warranted. For example, Ternes, Woody, and Livingston (1987) described an 11-year-old boy with atypical depressive features, academic deficits, and interpersonal difficulties associated with frequent right-temporal spikes on an electroencephalogram. He was treated with carbamazepine and showed a rapid response to his affective illness and interpersonal relations. After 1 year he did not present any recurrence of previous symptoms, and significant improvements in his previous academic deficits were observed.

Interventions at School

The school setting is particularly important because it is the environment where the main problems of children with NLD emerge and may also represent a crucial key for effective interventions. Moreover, it is the environment where children spend most of their time, thus psychological problems emerging at school and academic skill deficits are crucial to address. Improving competence in academically impaired areas may require some activities that occur at school (either individually or in the context of the classroom) and others that must be necessarily carried out within an extracurricular environment. For example, in 1997, the Padua lab (Cornoldi et al., 1997) published a large volume including activities developed for improving difficulties of children with NLD in the following areas:

- Visuospatial memory and visuospatial abilities
- Drawing
- Handwriting
- Arithmetic
- Geography
- Science
- Social skills

Table 7.2 presents some compensatory instruments that can be used by teachers based on the child's characteristics and the academic areas of difficulty. In general, given that one of the strength areas of children with NLD is represented by verbal abilities, teachers should encourage these children to use verbal strategies when visuospatial material is presented. There are curricula available in North America that take a verbal or narrative approach to mathematics—for example, Life of Fred Mathematics (Schmidt, 2011) uses simple but entertaining stories to teach mathematics from elementary to university levels covering calculus and statistics. Other approaches to mathematics emphasize mental calculation, teaching concepts without a strong writing demand. One example of this type of approach is the Verbal Math Lesson series that covers basic mathematics concepts, fractions, and percentages (Levin & Langton, 2007).

Teacher-modeled problem solving is important for teaching students with NLD. This method—also called cognitive apprenticeship—is based on the observation of an expert working on a task (Collins, Brown, & Newman, 1989) through verbal mediation or "think out loud." In particular, teaching methods that integrate spatial and verbal processes are useful in helping students to integrate their verbal strengths with their areas of weakness. For example, in drawing a figure, the child may improve his or her performance by verbally describing the figure prior to and while drawing it. Similarly, in order to improve the ability to put numbers in columns to perform written calculations, children may be helped first by consulting simple written instructions and then by using verbal self-instructions (see Van Luit, 2009). Often, children with NLD encounter difficulties in interpreting tables, figures, and graphs. For this reason tables and graphs should be described verbally in order to help children to integrate the presented information. In addition, children with NLD may not be helped by conceptual maps or diagrams for studying written materials—for improving their study method, teachers should suggest summaries and keywords instead of conceptual maps (Mammarella & Lipparini, 2015). In summary, teaching explicit and systematic cognitive strategies may be useful for children with NLD. Teachers may suggest that the child writes down strategies that were previously successful so that he or she can refer to these strategies when needed.

Another crucial role of the school is to cope with social interaction problems of children with NLD—shyness and social isolation may occur, as well as social rejection or bullying by their peers (Tanguay, 2001). Young children and preadolescents may meet difficulties in interacting with classmates and in particular with groups of children of the same age and of the same gender, looking for exclusive dual relationships or for interactions with groups of different ages. In adolescence, the problem may also be complicated by the child's difficulty in interacting with peers of the opposite sex. However, friendships with others are important for children with NLD. Teachers can take a leading role in creating supervised situations where the child interacts with other children. Despite the fact that researchers have not specifically considered the case of NLD, there is robust evidence that supervised peer tutoring and cooperative learning may be effective with children with social or learning difficulties (Jordan & Métais, 1997; Goodwin, 1999). Other useful strategies include giving specific responsibilities within the learning community to the child with NLD (Lavoie, 1994). Examples of this might include being a timekeeper and participating in organized groups such as collaborating for the class or school newspaper.

Finally, the school must support making decisions on the school curriculum that the child with NLD should follow. In many countries, vocational guidance is also an assumed responsibility of the school. Guidance that takes care to understand the individual strengths and weaknesses of children with NLD is important in guiding them to vocations aligned with their interests as well as their skills.

Interventions with the Family

Parenting stress is an important variable to consider when providing intervention to families (McDowell, Saylor, Taylor, Boyce, & Stokes, 1995). In particular, mothers with high levels of stress appear to be more controlling and punitive than mothers who have lower levels of stress (Webster-Stratton, 1990). In the case of developmental disabilities, several variables have been found to moderate parenting stress. Socioeconomic status is inversely related to levels of parenting stress (Kazdin, Stolar, & Marciano, 1995), boys are perceived as more stressful than girls, older children are perceived as more stressful for parents, and older parents seem to present with higher levels of stress than younger parents (Tunali & Power, 1993; Antshel & Joseph, 2006). In addition, single-parent households appear more likely to report higher levels of parenting stress (Thompson, Auslander, & White, 2001) when children are developmentally disabled in some way.

It is worth noting that high levels of parenting stress may be associated with increases in maternal depression (Hassiotis, 1997; Lipman, Offord, Dooley, & Boyle, 2002; Margalit, Raviv, & Ankonina, 1992; Moes, Koegel, Schreibman, & Loos, 1992). In 2006, Antshel and Joseph compared parental stress in mothers of children between 8 and 11 years old with a diagnosis of reading disorders (RD) or NLD. Mothers of children with RD reported higher levels of general distress while mothers of children with NLD reported higher levels of dysfunctional interactions with their child. The severity of the LD was strongly associated with maternal stress only in the sample of children with NLD. In this sample, the most powerful predictors of maternal stress were the presence in the child of low nonverbal IQ scores and the presence of internalizing symptoms. In the sample of children with RD, the strongest predictors of maternal stress were the age of the mother, her level of reported psychiatric symptoms, and her overall level of social support.

It is important to note, too, that there is evidence that stress experienced by the parent of developmentally disabled children decreases with effective treatment, even when parental stress is not the focus of the intervention (Kazdin & Wassell, 2000). Families can be supported and advised in a series of problems they may meet with children with NLD or that children may present within the family context. Based on different reports, Davis and Broitman (2011) mention a series of health risks of which parents should be aware. They mention, for example, the risk of injuries related with poor attention and motor coordination, and the risk of weight increase due to a sedentary life. Hence, according to Davis and Broitman (2011), child variables within the family context must also be considered when suggesting interventions for families involving children with NLD.

Although training programs designed specifically for parents of children with NLD are not available, there are good reasons for expecting that parent training could be as useful as it has been for other clinical groups. In particular, support programs for parents of children with similar symptoms such as ADHD, ASD, or LD are likely to benefit parents of children with NLD (see, e.g., Chronis, Chacko, Fabiano, Wymbs, & Pelham, 2004). Some of the common themes in parent training include basic psychoeducation on neurodevelopmental disorders, how to recognize critical issues, coping strategies, increasing consistency and authoritative parenting practices, coping with educational issues, and sharing family problems with other families that have similar situations.

A child's social isolation and dependency on parents can be a typical family problem. Parents may need help understanding how to positively approach promoting an active self-help role for their child. Direct instruction on how to develop and refine the social skills necessary for meaningful social relationships and interactions may be required. Through modeling, reinforcements, creation of useful opportunities, and providing direct instruction parents may help the child to progress socially. External positive reinforcements are sometimes necessary. When the child manifests appropriate social skills during everyday life, immediate encouragement should be tied to performance. It is also important for the child to perceive the social interaction as meaningful. Appropriate reinforcement may also promote peer recognition, and, more importantly, may maintain the child's motivation to interact with other people. It may be useful for the child with NLD to practice social interaction followed by introspection and reflection on the mental states of him- or herself and the others in the interaction. Drama- and performance-based games supporting the imitation of facial expressions and social role-playing may be similarly helpful along with journaling to foster reflection and utilize the verbal processing of these activities. A journal could include pictures, emotions, a list of situations encountered, dialogue, and the reflections of the child about the experiences.

Some families may wish to engage a clinical psychologist who can offer parents emotional support and guidance about decisions, inform them about developmental expectations based on the child's characteristics, and encourage them to identify the child's areas of strength. Intervention at home may interest not only family members but also other people. For example, especially when schooling is limited to the morning hours, as it may happen in some countries, homework and afternoon activities can be supervised by a tutor who supports the child, avoiding a conflict-prone interaction between the parent and child over homework, thus favoring the development of the child's autonomy.

Conclusion

As extensively shown in the present chapter, the literature has not fully tested intervention studies for children with NLD and shows many limitations. Nevertheless, by considering both published studies and clinical experience, we have tried to summarize key concepts into general guidelines for the clinical intervention of children with NLD and, in addition, to illustrate different kinds of interventions that clinicians, educators, and parents might use with NLD by considering psychomotor, visuoperceptual deficits, arithmetic difficulties and social interaction weaknesses. Furthermore, a multimodal approach intervening not only on the child with NLD but also on school, family and social contexts has been suggested. The choice of the intervention should vary according to the individual characteristics of the child—such as age, severity of deficits, degree of functional impairment, and presence of preserved abilities—and of the family, by considering the degree of parenting stress, which has been shown as a crucial variable which influences dysfunctional interactions between parents and children with NLD.

CHAPTER EIGHT

Case Studies

In this chapter, we report the cases of three children with a clinical diagnosis of NLD in order to give an overview of the assessment and intervention procedures adopted or suggested to parents, teachers, and other clinicians. As mentioned previously, the variety of cases within the NLD population is large and each child has specific characteristics that make him or her unique. To give an idea of this variety we have selected cases of different ages and genders and also followed with different kinds of interventions.

Case 1: Marco

Marco is an 8-year-old boy, attending the third grade of primary school, who was referred by his teachers because of concern about his difficulties in handwriting. Marco is a healthy child without hearing or vision problems. He was born at 37 weeks of gestational age (weighing 2.75 kilograms) and his first independent steps and first words were at 14 and 12 months, respectively. As a preschooler he did not like to draw, had fine-motor difficulties in activities such as opening and closing buttons, and started to use a bike after 5 years. His preschool teachers also indicated that he had difficulty interacting with other children. At the end of preschool, Marco was enrolled in a public primary school. Family history did not present psychiatric problems or genetic/developmental syndromes.

Marco's teachers expressed concerns about his schooling. Specifically, they noted poor handwriting and chaotic management of space on paper—for example, in putting numbers in columns during dictation. Figure 8.1 presents a sample of handwriting from Marco's exercise book.

Observations during the Assessment

Marco talks comfortably about his school and his interests, with an adult-like presentation uncommon to a child of his age. He likes listening to classical singer–songwriters and reading books. He prefers to be alone but has one or two friends with similar interests. He speaks continuously and is curious about the assessment tasks, but he needs several breaks in which he speaks about everything and anything. Marco is aware of his handwriting difficulties and reports that he prefers oral recitation as a form of study and presentation compared with written communication.

Assessment Procedure

Table 8.1 presents the scores obtained by Marco on the standardized tests administered during the assessment phase. The results of the assessment revealed that Marco did not have problems

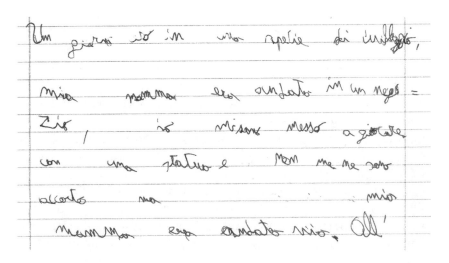

FIGURE 8.1. Example of handwriting taken from Marco's exercise book.

TABLE 8.1. Test Summary for Marco

Construct	Test	Standardized score
Reading decoding (reading of a passage)	*MT reading test* (Cornoldi & Colpo, 1998)	
	• Speed	$z = -0.63$
	• Accuracy (errors)	$z = 0.51$
Reading comprehension	*MT reading comprehension* (Cornoldi & Colpo, 1998)	
	• Accuracy	$z = 0.84$
Handwriting	*Writing fluency* (Tressoldi & Cornoldi, 1991)	
	• Subtest 1—speed	$z = -1.82$
	• Subtest 2—speed	$z = -2.66$
	• Subtest 3—speed	$z = -2.41$
	Writing production (Tressoldi, Cornoldi, & Re, 2012)	$z = -1.73$
Mathematics	*AC-MT battery* (Cornoldi, Lucangeli, & Bellina, 2012)	
	• Mental calculations	
	○ Errors	$z = 1.46$
	○ Speed	$z = -2.97$
	• Written calculations	
	○ Errors	$z = 1.50$
	○ Spccd	$z = -0.35$
	• Number dictation (errors)	$z > 3$
	• Numerical facts (errors)	$z = 0.65$
Visuoconstructive skills	*VMI* (Beery & Buktenica, 2006)	
	• Visual motor integration	**Standard score = 75**
	• Motor coordination	Standard score = 86
	Rey Complex Figure Test (Rey, 1967)	
	• Copy	$z < -3$
	• Recall	$z = -2.89$
Visuospatial working memory	*VSWM battery* (Mammarella et al., 2008b)	
	• Corsi blocks forward	$z = -0.39$
	• Corsi blocks backward	$z = -1.9$
	• Meaningless shapes	$z = -1.53$
	• Water animal recognition	$z = -0.61$

(continued)

TABLE 8.1. (continued)

Construct	Test	Standardized score
Visuospatial working memory (cont.)	• Balloons recognition	$z = -0.48$
	• Sequential light bulbs	$z = -0.56$
	• Sequential lines	$z = -1.37$
	• Sequential dots	**$z = -2.23$**
	• Simultaneous light bulbs	$z = -1.12$
	• Simultaneous lines	$z = -1.29$
	• Simultaneous dots	$z = 0.28$
	• Jigsaw puzzle	**$z = -2.64$**
	• Pathway span	**$z = -2.31$**
	• Active Visual Pattern Test	**$z = -1.74$**
Fine-motor skills	NEPSY-II (Korkman et al., 2007)	
	• Fingertip tapping	**Standard score = 5**
	• Imitating hand positions	**Standard score = 3**
General intelligence	WISC-IV (Wechsler, 2003)	
	• Full Scale IQ	104
	• Verbal Comprehension Index	132
	• Perceptual Reasoning Index	**85**
	• Working Memory Index	106
	• Processing Speed Index	**82**

Note. **Bold type** indicates particularly low scores.

either in reading decoding or in reading comprehension. However, his handwriting was laborious, and required a lot of effort; it took him more time than his same-age peers to write syllables and words.

In a writing production test (Tressoldi, Cornoldi, & Re, 2013), Marco was asked to describe some drawings depicting a story of a dog going with a child to school. Figure 8.2 presents his text production.

Marco's writing production is of poor quality and quite abbreviated (see English translation in the caption to Figure 8.2). However, when we asked Marco to orally describe the story depicted in the images he was more adequately descriptive. He said,

> It's autumn, since there are the leaves on the ground. There is a child playing with his dog. The dog says "hello" to the child

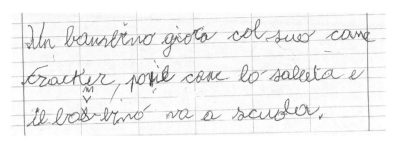

FIGURE 8.2. Marco's performance on the writing production test (Tressoldi et al., 2012) The text Marco produced includes some errors and a limited series of elements (translation: "A child plays with his dog named Cracker, then the dog greets him and the child goes to school").

who is going to school, also if he would prefer to play again. The dog is sad, because he is alone out of the school.

Thus, Marco was able to produce a nice story, to observe some details (mentioning the leaves on the ground), and to make inferences about the emotional state of the characters (he reports that the dog is sad, because he is alone outside of the school). When we asked Marco why he did not write all these details, he answered that handwriting requires too much effort for him.

In the math achievement task (Cornoldi Lucangeli, & Bellina, 2012), Marco's performance was poor, both in speed and accuracy in performing mental calculations. In addition, he made several errors on written calculations (see Figure 8.3). In the number dictation task, Marco was required to write numbers dictated by the experimenter and he made a lot of mistakes. On the contrary, he had no problems in recalling arithmetic facts.

Marco performed poorly on both the VMI and the Rey Complex Figure Test; Figure 8.4 presents his drawings on the Rey. As discussed in Chapter 6, in the copy phase, the examinee has to copy a meaningless complex figure, while in the recall phase, the examinee has to remember the figure after a few minutes and then draw it. Marco followed an unusual way to draw the figure, as it was possible to reconstruct from the different colors used. He began his reproduction without drawing the rectangular pattern with diagonals although he did observe and reproduce the details of the complex figure. In the recall

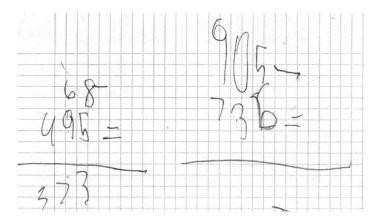

FIGURE 8.3. Example of Marco's written calculations.

phase, he followed the same strategy, but lost some elements and in particular, he did not remember the relationship among the various details. The heavier lines in Figure 8.4 indicate the parts Marco drew with the first two colors. It may be seen that, when starting the drawing, he did not have the overall organization of the figure in mind, and in particular, did not reproduce the rectangle as a unitary pattern, in contrast to how the majority of children perform.

On the VSWM battery (Mammarella et al., 2008b) Marco failed all the active tasks, requiring not only to remember but also to manipulate visuospatial information. His performance on the Corsi backward task was also poor and he obtained low scores on both tasks taken from the NEPSY-II battery (Korkman et al., 2011) to assess fine-motor skills. Finally, Marco's IQ was measured using the WISC-IV (Wechsler, 2003). A specific pattern of results emerged. In particular, he performed above average on the Verbal Comprehension Index (VCI) (with a VCI score of 132, two standard deviations above the normative mean score) and below average on the Perceptual Reasoning Index (PRI) (with a PRI score of 85). More specifically, Marco performed poorly on the Block Design and Matrix Reasoning subtests compared with his better performances on Vocabulary and Comprehension; his processing speed was slow compared with other children of his age. In sum, Marco met all the criteria for a diagnosis of NLD

Copy

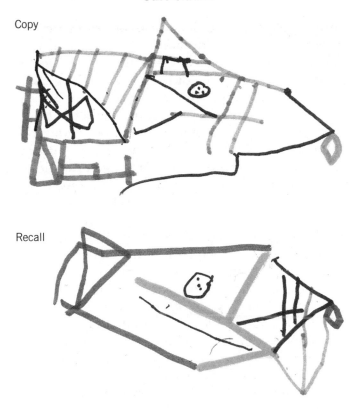

Recall

FIGURE 8.4. The Complex Figure test drawn by Marco. (The heavier lines indicate the parts Marco drew using the first two colors.)

and appeared particularly poor in a series of cognitive (visuospatial) and academic (writing and mathematics) areas.

Intervention

Marco received a specialized intervention in our service for LD at the University of Padua. In particular, 16 training sessions were developed with the following goals:

- Improve fine-motor skills and handwriting.
- Improve expressive writing skills.
- Improve VSWM.

These three goals were considered as priorities for Marco on the basis of a series of considerations. In particular, we tried to develop handwriting in order to make him more effective when writing and to take advantage of his good oral language expressive skills for use in writing. In fact, we considered an improvement in written text production within Marco's high potential, but also felt that this improvement should be further promoted by teaching some basic skills underlying text production. Obviously, Marco presented with a broader range of difficulties, but because we only had a limited number of sessions we preferred to focus on writing and on a more general cognitive component (VSWM) that represented a particularly relevant area of weakness. In discussing the program with Marco's family, we decided to focus on three well-defined and partly related aspects, leaving the other aspects to a successive intervention.

In order to improve handwriting and fine-motor skills, exercises with a pen–tablet device were proposed. The device consists of a flat surface upon which the examinee draws or writes by using an attached stylus, a pen-like drawing apparatus in which the image representing his or her production is displayed on a computer monitor. These kinds of exercises require high oculomanual coordination, but also involve the development of a mental representation of the graphic production and thus allow improvement of both graphic trait and speed, and the underlying representations guiding hand production. In order to improve writing production, Marco was trained in metacognitive and control skills devoted to developing self-efficacy and self-confidence in writing and improving the abilities in generating ideas and planning the order in which ideas could be arranged in a text. Finally, to improve VSWM, a computerized program was used (Mammarella et al., 2010b). In particular, Marco was presented with the active VSWM section of the computerized program, in which he was involved in tasks that required not only maintaining but also processing and manipulating visuospatial information.

As shown in Table 8.2, Marco improved in all areas of the intervention. His handwriting performance, when not completely averaged for speed, also showed a significant improvement. Figure 8.5 presents the writing fluency test before and after the intervention. As can be seen, in the same quantity of time (1 minute for each of the three phases), Marco was able to write more and more letters than before the intervention. His writing production appeared to be normalized at the end of the treatment. Hence, by reducing the effort and increasing speed and being guided in text production, Marco was able to take advantage of his good oral expressive skills.

Visuospatial memory showed an improvement after the intervention. In particular, in the active tasks on which we focused during the intervention, Marco obtained scores comparable with those of the normative sample for his age. The treatment and its effects were perceived and appreciated by his family and school and also by Marco himself.

TABLE 8.2. Results of the Intervention with Marco

Construct	Test	Pretraining performance	Posttraining performance
Handwriting	*Writing fluency* (Tressoldi & Cornoldi, 1991)		
	• Subtest 1—speed	$z = \mathbf{-1.82}$	$z = -1.73$
	• Subtest 2—speed	$z = \mathbf{-2.66}$	$z = -0.97$
	• Subtest 3—speed	$z = \mathbf{-2.41}$	$z = -1.41$
	Writing production (Tressoldi et al., 2012)	$z = -1.37$	$z = 0.45$
Visuospatial working memory	*VSWM battery* (Mammarella et al., 2008b)		
	• Corsi blocks forward	$z = -0.39$	$z = 0.21$
	• Corsi blocks backward	$z = \mathbf{-1.9}$	$z = -0.58$
	• Meaningless shapes	$z = \mathbf{-1.53}$	$z = -0.47$
	• Water animal recognition	$z = -0.61$	$z = 0.04$
	• Balloons recognition	$z = -0.48$	$z = -0.12$
	• Sequential light bulbs	$z = -0.56$	$z = -0.25$
	• Sequential lines	$z = -1.37$	$z = -1.12$
	• Sequential dots	$z = \mathbf{-2.23}$	$z = -1.03$
	• Simultaneous light bulbs	$z = -1.12$	$z = -0.91$
	• Simultaneous lines	$z = -1.29$	$z = -0.89$
	• Simultaneous dots	$z = -0.28$	$z = 0.17$
	Jigsaw puzzle	$z = \mathbf{-2.64}$	$z = -0.21$
	• Pathway Span	$z = \mathbf{2.31}$	$z = -0.96$
	• Active Visual Pattern Test	$z = -1.74$	$z = -0.18$

Note. **Bold type** indicates particularly low scores.

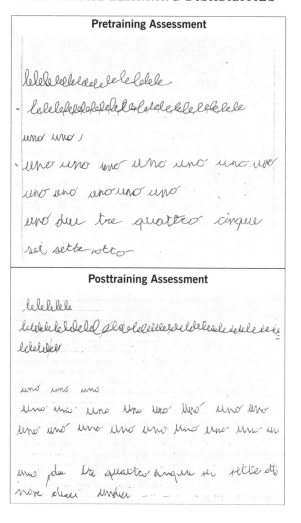

FIGURE 8.5. Marco's performance on the writing fluency test (Tressoldi & Cornoldi, 1991) before (top) and after (bottom) the intervention.

Case 2: Sofia

Sofia is a 13-year-old eighth-grade girl, who wears eyeglasses and braces on her teeth. Her mother is divorced; Sofia sees her father twice a month. Sofia received a previous diagnosis of social phobia with severe difficulties in mathematics when she was 7 years old. She was born at 38 weeks gestational age (weighing 3.15 kilograms) and her first independent steps and first words were at

15 and 13 months, respectively. As a preschooler she had fine-motor difficulties and was afraid to play with other children with balls and other toys that required coordination. She was also afraid of water and until age 10 did not learn how to swim. She started to use a bike at age 8 but worried about speed. Sofia's preschool teachers indicated that she had difficulties interacting with other children. However, she learned to read at 5 years of age; at the end of preschool, she was enrolled in a public primary school. Sofia developed asthma and was repeatedly hospitalized for bronchial pneumonia; her teachers expressed concerns about her poor mathematics achievement. Her family history was described as negative for psychiatric problems and genetic/developmental syndromes.

Observations during the Assessment

Sofia is a shy and quiet girl, who speaks only when she receives direct questions. She was a victim of bullying the year before our assessment and for this reason she changed schools. She reports that now the situation is better, and that she has established friendships with two girls. However, she likes to go out with her mom, or to stay at home watching TV or playing with her dog. Her best friend is a girl with a visual disability. Sofia is aware of her own difficulties, in particular, she tells us she is worried about oral exams and mathematics exercises; she feels anxious when she is in front of a blank sheet of paper.

Assessment Procedure

In Table 8.3 we present Sofia's scores that were obtained with standardized instruments administered during the assessment phase. The results of the assessment revealed that Sofia did not have problems in reading decoding. However, she showed weaknesses in reading comprehension and handwriting. Furthermore, in the mathematics achievement task (Cornoldi & Cazzola, 2003), Sofia was slower than her peers in performing calculations; in addition, she made several errors on written calculations due to column confusion (see Figure 8.6). She also obtained poor scores in retrieving arithmetic facts and in performing approximate calculations.

TABLE 8.3. Test Summary for Sofia

Construct	Test	Score
Reading decoding	*MT reading test* (Cornoldi & Colpo, 1998)	
	• Speed	$z = 0.10$
	• Accuracy	$z = 0.75$
Reading comprehension	*MT reading comprehension* (Cornoldi & Colpo, 1998)	
	• Accuracy	$z = -0.90$
Handwriting	*Writing fluency* (Tressoldi & Cornoldi, 1991)	
	• Subtest 1—speed	$z = -1.10$
	• Subtest 2—speed	$z = -1.27$
	• Subtest 3—speed	$z = -0.97$
	Writing production (Tressoldi et al., 2012)	$z = -1.35$
Mathematics	*AC-MT battery 11–14* (Cornoldi & Cazzola, 2003)	
	• Mental calculations	
	○ Errors	$z = 0.15$
	○ Speed	$z = 2.78$
	• Written calculations	
	○ Errors	$z = 1.35$
	○ Speed	$z > 3.00$
	• Number dictation (errors)	$z = 0.36$
	• Numerical facts (errors)	$z = 2.56$
	• Approximate calculation (errors)	$z = 1.93$
Visuoconstructive skills	*VMI* (Beery & Buktenica, 2006)	
	• Visual motor integration	**Standard score = 65**
	• Motor coordination	Standard score = 88
	Rey Complex Figure Test (Rey, 1967)	
	• Copy	$z = -2.92$
	• Recall	$z = -2.52$
Visuospatial working memory	*VSWM battery* (Mammarella et al., 2008b)	
	• Corsi blocks forward	$z = -0.95$
	• Corsi blocks backward	$z = -1.78$

(continued)

TABLE 8.3. *(continued)*

Construct	Test	Score
Visuospatial working memory *(cont.)*	• Jigsaw puzzle • Pathway Span • Active Visual Pattern Test	$z = -1.46$ $z = -1.81$ $z = -0.49$

Fine-motor skills	*NEPSY-II* (Korkman et al., 2007)
	  • Fingertip tapping
	  • Imitating hand positions
		
		Standard score = 7
		Standard score = 1

Anxiety	*SAFA self-questionnaire* (Cianchetti & Sannio Fancello, 2001)
	  • General anxiety
	  • Social anxiety
	  • Separation anxiety
	  • School anxiety
		
		$T = 61$
		$T = 73$
		$T = 38$
		$T = 48$

Self-esteem	*Multidimensional Self Concept Scale* (Bracken, 1992)
	  • Interpersonal self-esteem
	  • Scholastic self-esteem
	  • Family self-esteem
	  • Physics self-esteem
		
		$T = 51$
		$T = 61$
		$T = 65$
		$T = 66$

General intelligence	*WISC-IV* (Wechsler, 2003)
	  • Full Scale IQ
	  • Verbal Comprehension Index
	  • Perceptual Reasoning Index
	  • Working Memory Index
	  • Processing Speed Index
		
		90
		120
		85
		79
		76

Note. **Bold type** indicates particularly low scores.

Sofia performed poorly on both the VMI and the Rey Complex Figure Test. Figure 8.7 presents Sofia's performance on some items of the VMI, in which she also encountered difficulties in copying simple figures—for example, she was not able to maintain the size of the shapes and their spatial relationships.

We only administered active tasks from the VSWM battery (Mammarella et al., 2008b); Sofia performed poorly on two of three subtests and the Corsi Block task, where she had particular difficulty with backward recall. In both tasks taken from the NEPSY-II battery (Korkman et al., 2007) to assess fine-motor

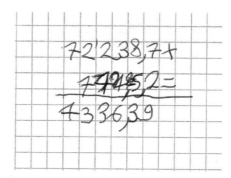

FIGURE 8.6. Example of Sofia's written calculations (the required operation is 72238.7 – 712.52).

skills, she demonstrated poor development. Due to emotional problems reported during the intake interview, Sofia was presented with two questionnaires: the first analyzed her anxiety and the latter her self-esteem. Results showed high scores on general, social, and separation anxiety; she also reported low self-esteem in the areas of school, family, and physical aspects. Finally, Sofia's IQ was measured using the WISC-IV (Wechsler, 2003), where a specific pattern of results emerged. In particular, she performed above average on the VCI (i.e., VCI score of 120) and below average on the PRI (i.e., PRI score of 85). In addition, she obtained low scores on processing speed and WM indices. In sum, Sofia met the criteria for the diagnosis of NLD with a high discrepancy between verbal and nonverbal intelligence,

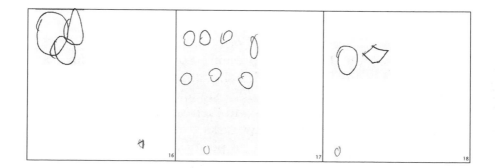

FIGURE 8.7. Some examples taken from the VMI test made by Sofia.

including low visuospatial skills and weaknesses in mathematics, motor coordination, and social aspects.

Intervention

In Sofia's case, the University Center in Padua was involved only in the diagnosis and proposed intervention because she was followed by a clinician and teachers in her town. To define priorities for Sofia, we considered her profile, age, and available resources. In particular, we considered the fact that Sofia was an adolescent experiencing severe adaptive consequences due to her social difficulties. An improvement in mathematics was considered to be a reasonable goal given her generally good overall ability and its necessity for the continuation of her school career. Overall, she appeared intelligent, reflective, and willing to better understand herself, but in need of more motivation. Therefore, we suggested the following areas of intervention:

- A specific program to improve social abilities and reduce social anxiety. Sofia should be helped to understand emotions in herself and in others and control them in order to improve social interactions with peers. Parallel with the clinical intervention, teachers should support Sofia's self-esteem and motivation at school by structuring activities and facilitating social interactions with her classmates. Both teachers and parents should acknowledge her success in any academic field in order to avoid a further reduction in academic self-confidence.

- An intensive intervention on mathematics abilities. The intervention should focus on developing verbal strategies to help Sofia cope with her visuospatial problems in written calculation. In addition, complex tasks should be divided into different steps toward reaching the final goal by consolidating (with the development of awareness and with repeated practice) the basic arithmetic operations that involve visuospatial processes (e.g., number writing, columns). When word problems are presented at school, a calculator could be given to Sofia so that she can avoid mistakes due to wrong calculations.

- In general, Sofia should be assisted in gaining a better understanding of her own strengths and weaknesses, in developing motivation and perceptions of self-efficacy, and in using verbal strategies and self-instructions toward coping with her academic difficulties.

Case 3: Daniel

Daniel is a left-handed 15-year-old boy who was referred to a neuropsychological center in the United States by his pediatrician with concerns about anxiety and learning. Recently, Daniel had been experiencing panic attacks and appeared to be withdrawing from friends and family. He lives with his parents, both of whom are college-educated white-collar professionals. An older brother lives away from home and attends a high-level Ivy League college. There is a family history of giftedness and mathematics learning problems. Daniel engages in a wide range of intellectual and creative activities, including playing violin with the school orchestra.

Daniel was born healthy following a full-term unremarkable pregnancy and birth. His parents reported that he was easily soothed and well regulated for sleeping and eating, but that his temperament was shy and risk aversive as a toddler. He preferred to sit and watch rather than join in "rough-and-tumble" play in the park with other children. Motor milestones were met within broadly typical limits; walking was mildly delayed at 18 months. Expressive and receptive language skills were noted as precocious, with five-word complex sentences emerging at about 2 years of age. Daniel learned to read at about 4 years old, prior to entering elementary school.

No problems were reported either academically or socially during most of elementary school. During his fifth-grade year, Daniel encountered problems in mathematics. A tutor was engaged three times per week to help him learn long division and complex multiplication. There was a period of increased anxiety during the transition to middle school that included transient tics and lack of appetite, and mathematics learning problems persisted. Daniel began to engage in negative self-talk regarding his ability to learn, saying often that he was "the stupid one in the family." Up until this point Daniel read widely for pleasure, but since the eighth grade he had difficulty with reading comprehension for higher-level history and English literature subjects. His parents reported that he has excellent spelling skills, but difficulty gaining insight and developing ideas for demanding comprehensive written projects. Daniel reported that he has difficulty taking notes during lectures so he does not bother. He understands the lectures but cannot recall the information when he gets home, so he does not perform well on in-class exams. He is currently failing mathematics and history.

Observations during the Assessment

Daniel presented as friendly but mildly shy. Eye contact was observed as normal. His spoken language was fluent, with normal prosody and age-appropriate vocabulary and pragmatic conversational skills. He demonstrated excellent perseverance and focus during the assessment. No overt signs of performance anxiety were noted.

Assessment Procedure

The assessment plan included evaluation to rule out anxiety disorder; specific LD in mathematics without NLD (e.g., executive function or verbal mathematics deficits); NLD; ADHD, inattentive subtype, with global memory and executive problems; and mild ASD. The assessment comprised a parent interview; a child interview; clinical observation of behaviors during testing; information gathered from teachers; rating scales of mood, executive functioning behaviors; and academic and social functioning from parents, teachers, and Daniel; as well as direct testing of specific neuropsychological processes, including intellectual development (verbal/language—reduced), motor, visuomotor integration, visual scanning, memory (verbal/visual, contextual/abstract, simple/complex), sustained attention, planning and organizational skill, mental flexibility, verbal fluency, and strategy development (see Table 8.4).

The alternative hypothesis of ASD was ruled out via intake interview and Daniel's presentation. ADHD was ruled out via rating scales and direct observation via the Test of Variables

TABLE 8.4. Test Summary for Daniel

Construct	Test	Score
Intellectual development	*WISC-IV* (Wechsler, 2003) • Verbal Comprehension • Perceptual Reasoning	*SS* = 116 *SS* = 94
Motor-planning/ speed	*Lafayette Grooved Pegs* (Larson, Kirschner, Bode, Heinemann, & Goodman, 2005)	Left (dom) z = –1.2 Right z = –1.0
Visuomotor integration	*VMI* (Beery & Buktenica, 2006)	*SS* = 84
	VMI (perceptual)	**SS = 85**
	RCFT copy (Osterrieth, 1944)	**%ile 3–10**
	WISC-IV Coding	*SS* = 8
Visual scanning	*WISC-IV Symbol Search*	*SS* = 8 (due to errors)
	D-KEFS Trails: 1. Visual Scanning (Delis et al., 2001)	*SS* = 8 (accurate but slow)
Auditory memory	*WISC-IV Working Memory Index*	*SS* = 105
	CVLT-C word list learning (Delis et al., 1994)	Trial 1: z = –1, Trial 5: z = 0 Semantic recall: z = 0.5 Delayed free: z = 0.5
	WRAML Story Memory (Sheslow & Adams, 2003)	*SS* = 10
Visual memory	*WISC-IV Integrated Corsi Block*	**SS = 7**
	RCFT Immediate/Delayed Recall (Osterrieth, 1944)	*T* = 45/**38**
	WRAML Design Memory (Sheslow & Adams, 2003)	**SS = 7**
	WRAML Picture Memory (Sheslow & Adams, 2003)	*SS* = 8
Academic reading	*TOWRE-2 Sight Words* (Torgesen et al., 1999)	*SS* = 112
	TOWRE Pseudo Words (Torgesen et al., 2012)	*SS* = 120
	GORT-5 (Wiederholt & Bryant, 2012)	Fluency = 14 Comprehension = 11

(continued)

TABLE 8.4. *(continued)*

Construct	Test	Score
Academic mathematics	*Key Math–3* (Connolly, 2007) • Numeration • Algebra • Geometry • Measurement • Data Analysis and Probability • Addition and Subtraction • Multiplication and Division • Applied Problem Solving	*SS* = **7** *SS* = 8 *SS* = 9 *SS* = 8 *SS* = 8 *SS* = 8 *SS* = **7** *SS* = **7**
Sustained attention	*TOVA* (McCarney & Greenberg, 1990)	Low probability ADHD match
Planning/ sequencing	*D-KEFS Trails* (Delis et al., 2001)	Trail 2. Numbers: *SS* = 9 Trail 3. Letters: *SS* = 10
Mental flexibility	*D-KEFS Trails* (Delis et al., 2001)	Trail 4. Switching: *SS* = 8 FAS: *SS* = 12
	D-KEFS Verbal Fluency (Delis et al., 2001)	Category: *SS* = 11 Switching: *SS* = 11
Strategy development	*CVLT-C Semantic Ratio* (Delis et al., 1994) • Testing observations	Serial z = 1.5 Semantic z = **–2.0** Difficulty changing strategies on Block Design and other visual tasks; tended to use a "hit-or-miss" approach
Behavioral executive functioning	*BRIEF Parent, Teacher, Self* (Gioia, Isquith, Guy, & Kenworthy, 2000)	Clinically significant elevations on Organization of Materials; otherwise, all other scales within typical range
Psychosocial functioning	*BASC-2 Parent, Teacher, Self* (Reynolds & Kamphaus, 2004)	School-related anxiety
	Child interview	Social anxiety as peers are high achieving, while Daniel is falling behind; fear regarding college, low self-esteem, uncertain future

Note. **Bold type** indicates particularly low scores.

of Attention (TOVA; McCarney & Greenberg, 1990). Daniel demonstrated well-developed verbal skills overall, especially in decoding and verbal concept formation. His WISC-IV Perceptual Reasoning Index was not below average, rather it was at the lower end of the average range. However, in concert with much stronger language-based reasoning; poor motor, visuomotor integration, and visuoperception problems (see Figure 8.8.); delayed mathematics skills; and mode-specific memory challenges for visual information compared with verbal, Daniel's profile aligned well with NLD. Error analyses of basic mathematics calculation indicated difficulty with decimals, orders of magnitude, multiplication, and division (see Figure 8.9). During the assessment, it became clear that Daniel had particular difficulty with visuoperception and memory. Although he demonstrated typical auditory memory for short, discrete stimuli, he had difficulty organizing complex auditory information that was highly contextual. Although he could recall as much as others, his method was concrete rather than conceptually based. Daniel appeared to have some difficulty when presented with large amounts of information that was not "preorganized" for him. However, he responded to direct instruction in strategy, as was observed on his recall improvement for words following categorical clustering on the California Verbal Learning Test (CVLT-C; Delis et al., 1994).

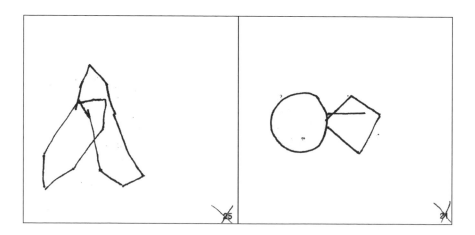

FIGURE 8.8. Daniel's copying of simple figures.

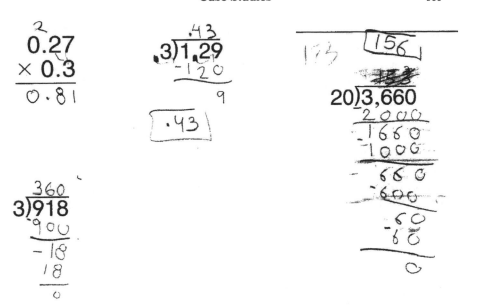

FIGURE 8.9. Sample of Daniel's mathematics calculation errors, which show confusion of decimal/order of magnitude and difficulty with long division.

Intervention

The intervention plan was focused on providing support for Daniel's weaknesses in the form of environmental accommodations and modifications to reduce barriers to learning. These included preferential seating at the front of the class; verbal instructions; keyboard training to facilitate note taking; and use of an integrated system (Smartpen) for synchronization of lecture, board, and notes. It was recommended that teacher Powerpoint presentations and lecture notes be provided to Daniel prior to lectures, if possible. Because Daniel had passed the age where handwriting is taught, it was recommended that all of his written products be computer based or dictated, even for exams. Academic coaching was to be focused not only on mathematics, but on *metacognitive* skills and critical reading strategies to help Daniel develop better memory of complex information, such as history and complex literature. A verbal approach to mathematics coaching was suggested, along with critical metacognitive procedures on how to estimate reasonable order of magnitude for error checking in mathematic procedures. Book chapters and articles for Daniel, his parents, academic coach, and teachers were provided, including a reference for a verbal mathematics approach and memory skills. An incentive system for developing keyboarding skills over the summer was proposed.

Psychoeducation about NLD for Daniel, his family, and his school was undertaken so that Daniel could learn to advocate for himself with the support of others. Consultation regarding appropriate steps to college and college fit were discussed. The assessment itself proved therapeutic because Daniel was fully able to understand that his problem was not a matter of intellectual ability, but rather a specific difference in the way he learns. However, it was suggested that Daniel learn some methods for reducing anxiety via psychological counseling if, after implementing accommodations, his anxiety persisted. It was suggested that Daniel continue to be encouraged to find activities at which he could excel outside of school to confer psychological resilience.

Epilogue

In conclusion, NLD represents an important, promising, and stimulating aspect of developmental clinical psychology. We hope that readers will now be able to share the emotions we experienced when we initiated our research and clinical practice with children with NLD. At that time, we immediately realized that we were exploring a world with distinct psychological characteristics and a deep need for additional research and empirically guided treatment. This book synthesizes the work carried out by us and by other researchers and clinicians working throughout the world. We have found that there exists a relevant body of research on NLD, larger than expected and quite independent from the work of the pioneers in the field.

As noted in the previous chapters, skepticism about NLD does not concern the existence of the problem, but rather its definition and the apparent lack of coherent evidence. We suggest that such skepticism is attributable to a partial knowledge of the literature; the common discussion is based primarily on the original work of only a few authors. As our updated reviews of the literature show, there is converging evidence that a constellation of neuropsychological characteristics and associated problems constitute the core features of NLD, whereas other features that are sometimes referred to in children with NLD are not necessarily present, resulting in substantial confusion in the field.

A related element of confusion is the association of NLD with other clinical categories that share some of its characteristics.

This may also explain why some people do not consider NLD to be a distinct diagnostic category; they assume that using extant diagnoses will mitigate the proliferation of clinical labels. However, this position appears to be particularly dangerous, as it incorrectly emphasizes isolated features associated with NLD (e.g., difficulties with mathematics, motor coordination, social relationships) and ignores other associated problems. We have assessed children with NLD who had previously received such diagnoses as developmental dyscalculia or dysgraphia, DCD, ASD, and ADHD. These earlier diagnoses often resulted in confusion and embarrassment among the families, the teachers, and the children themselves. Imagine a boy with minor communicative and relational problems, associated with the typical symptoms of NLD, being diagnosed with AS or HFA. The family receives painful news, and teachers and clinicians implement standard treatment for ASD. The boy may be required to participate in programs specific to autism when in fact, if well monitored and supported, he could manage everyday life much better than his autistic peers. Now imagine a girl with NLD being diagnosed with an LD such as dysgraphia who subsequently receives a handwriting intervention, ignoring the other challenges she faces in visuospatial abilities, mathematics, or social tasks. A more thorough description of her characteristics, including the NLD profile, would better detail her needs and developmental trajectory, and inform selection of an intervention program. Hence, if in general we agree that proliferation of clinical categories should be avoided, then the parsimony afforded by a correct diagnosis is that much more important.

We hope that some points have been clarified by our survey of the field, but we agree that other issues remain open and require further research in the future. Certainly some confusion about the NLD profile and the absence of explicit and consistent criteria have limited systematic research in the field. Some researchers, including ourselves, have already proposed diagnostic criteria for NLD, but the field had not reached a level a maturity to support robust direction. However, we now believe that the knowledge base has developed sufficiently to offer more reliable guidance. If our conclusions are at least partly shared by the scientific and clinical communities, it may soon be possible to fill the many gaps in the actual body of knowledge. The issue of intervention, in particular, appears at the moment to be inadequately addressed, with little confirmation of evidence-based efficacy regarding treatment. A second area in need of attention is epidemiological studies, which should strengthen the argument to add NLD to the diagnostic classification systems.

In the pages that follow, we try to summarize the main points delineated in this book as well as areas of NLD research that seem especially in need of further investigation.

The argument for the existence of NLD has historical precedent.

• *Models of psychological and neural functioning have always recognized the importance of within-person variations between verbal and nonverbal functioning.* The main theories of intelligence—both basic (e.g., Vernon, 1964) and related to assessment (e.g., Wechsler, 1991) and to the classical neuropsychological approaches (e.g., Nichelli & Venneri, 1995)—have all depicted cognition as distinct in at least these two aspects. Most cognitive batteries include subtests that distinguish between verbal and nonverbal processing, while many other widely used instruments measure more narrow, nonverbal cognitive processes (Evers et al., 2012). The concept of hemispheric specialization is also anchored in the verbal versus nonverbal contrast. Examples of nonverbal aspects include visual, spatial, and motor psychological processes. Nonverbal characteristics have also been recognized as contributing to social and emotional development (Rourke, 1995) in addition to reasoning, memory, and visuomotor integration.

• *Nonverbal characteristics appear highly related to one another, and also to the NLD syndrome, and justify their specification as part of the NLD label.* For example, strong evidence supports the relationship between different spatial and visual processes (e.g., Bunton & Fogarty, 2003; Logie, 1995) but also between visuospatial memory and motor coordination (Alloway & Archibald, 2008).

• *It is common to find weaknesses in nonverbal functioning among children.* Surveys of clinicians in different countries report the frequent presence of children with a series of nonverbal difficulties (e.g., Solodow et al., 2006).

• *The development of procedures for and clinical descriptions of nonverbal weaknesses has been documented in several places around the world,* suggesting that the profile may be universal, and the NLD profile is considered relevant in many countries. It is interesting to note that several important tests used to assess nonverbal functioning have their origins in different countries. For example, the Bender–Gestalt test from Germany (Bender, 1946) has been widely used in its American adaptations (e.g., Beery & Buktenica, 2006); the Rey Complex Figure Test (Rey, 1941) comes from the French-speaking tradition; the Corsi test (Corsi, 1972) was developed in Canada; and the working memory batteries come from both British (e.g., Alloway, Gathercole, & Pickering, 2006) and Italian (Mammarella et al., 2008b) contexts.

• *The prevalence of the NLD diagnostic category internationally supports the existence of the profile.* Not only are problems typically associated with NLD often reported in the clinical descriptions of children, but specific reference to the NLD label is very often present (Johnson & Myklebust, 1967; Rourke, 1989; Solodow et al., 2006).

The diagnostic classification for NLD is currently in disarray, which may harm children and families, and is in need of evidence-based cohesion; nevertheless, it appears necessary.

• *The main diagnostic classification systems recognize the existence of NLD in a piecemeal rather than holistic manner.* Weaknesses in functioning can be described within the domains of motor coordination, or mathematics, or nonverbal communication, without considering that these aspects are often present together. Moreover, scarce attention is paid to the visual and spatial aspects. It is interesting to note that some descriptions of these clinical profiles include elements that refer to the NLD profile. For example, the description offered by ICD-10 (World Health Organization, 1992) of adolescents with DCD emphasizes the presence of visuospatial problems.

• *The profile of NLD, as proposed by different authors, has captured the characteristic strengths and weaknesses of NLD and offers a description of their relatedness.* In contrast to the single-symptom diagnoses most typically associated with children with NLD (e.g., LD, HFA), a diagnosis of NLD by definition includes the co-occurrence of related characteristics.

• *The NLD profile has been associated with a series of serious adaptive problems that should not be overlooked despite problems with the diagnostic category.* An important problem of NLD is that the adaptive consequences may be particularly severe and increase with age, in contrast with other specific LD, language disorders, or DCD, wherein problems mitigate with development (DSM-5; American Psychiatric Association, 2013). Ignoring or reducing to a narrow perspective the problems of children with NLD may result in serious consequences for their development and adaptation in adult life.

• *A serious consideration of the currently recognized neurodevelopmental disorders reveals that all of them presented problems for the definition of their characteristics and identification criteria prior to acceptance.* Most still maintain ambiguities and controversies. For example, the definition of LD, ADHD, or ASD have all met with ambiguities and modifications, changes in the diagnostic classification systems, and challenges as to how they should be conceptualized (see, e.g., the differences between DSM-1 [American Psychiatric Association, 1952] and DSM-5 [American Psychiatric Association, 2013]). The present status of the definition of NLD may be considered as an early stage of acceptance consistent with the history of other neurodevelopmental disorders.

The lack of clearly defined criteria has impeded both research and clinical applications, but consensus has begun to emerge.

• *Lacking an authoritative shared definition, differences in research sampling have made it difficult to compare diagnostic and intervention studies and to generalize findings.* The systematic presentation and comparison of studies, offered in the first chapters of this volume, exposes how the clinical groups of different studies were defined. There are many relevant discrepancies, both in the defining characteristics and outcomes.

• *Despite research discrepancies, there is now a relevant corpus of knowledge concerning children diagnosed as NLD and a systematic analysis of the literature can help in understanding NLD.* In fact, the number of studies that have considered NLD is rather impressive for a syndrome not officially recognized by the medical community. Part of the underestimation of relevant research is a result of the different labels that have historically been used for children with NLD (e.g., right-hemisphere developmental LD, visuo-spatial LD). Moreover, the literature appears in many different sources, among them academic, nursing, medical, and psychological journals.

• *The analysis of this corpus reveals that some principal diagnostic criteria may find substantial agreement between clinicians and researchers.* We are convinced that the majority of clinicians would agree with the diagnoses of NLD offered for single cases described in this book or in other sources, whereas some minor discrepancies would emerge in the consideration of exact criteria, as here proposed in Chapter 5. Yet, consensus is a necessary next step in research and clinical diagnoses.

• *The identification of not only shared criteria but also shared assessment procedures may help in developing comparable research and common practices in different countries around the world.* Some well-consolidated procedures are already available but should be integrated worldwide for both methodological and normative data. Because NLD symptoms are primarily nonverbal, it may be that the usual barriers of language and culture would not be as difficult to overcome as is with language-based disorders.

• *Shared criteria for NLD are needed to establish epidemiological research on the prevalence of the problem, the lack of such research presents a barrier to allocating resources to the population.* Epidemiological research is affected by the criteria adopted for a diagnosis. For example, DSM-5 (American Psychiatric Association, 2013) revised the criteria for the diagnosis of LD and ASD from those in DSM-IV-TR (American Psychiatric Association, 2000), and as a consequence the incidence and prevalence data should change. However, the absolute absence of data on the distribution of NLD creates serious problems, especially in allocation of resources. Concerning the frequency of cases with NLD, it should be noted that some research studies in the field were carried by by screening within the school population, but the percentages of NLD cases found in this way could substantially vary because of differences in study criteria.

• *Shared criteria for NLD should also offer the possibility to carry out systematic research on the neurobiological bases of NLD.* At this moment, research indicates that crucial brain areas associated with NLD can be identified (see Chapter 4). Future research should better develop the field-testing of emerging hypotheses on the role of these areas. The identification of clear criteria and the incidence of NLD will also give hope to a more systematic examination of the clinical anamnesis: the familywide presence of similar problems and/or neurobiological characteristics in the child's relatives.

Areas of research that deserve special attention include lifespan and treatment.

• *No clear evidence exists on the characteristics of NLD in adults and its consequences.* It is logical to assume that, given its neurobiological bases, the NLD profile and some associated problems would persist throughout the entire lifespan. In the preceding chapters, we have mentioned some supporting evidence, without dedicating specific attention to this issue. Rourke (1995) has suggested that the adaptive problems of individuals with NLD should increase, rather than attenuate, with age, which is a concern, but nonetheless unsubstantiated. It is also plausible to predict that some social, spatial, and intellectual weaknesses associated with the NLD profile may have serious consequences on adult life, but there is little evidence to guide our thinking on this as yet.

• *Children with NLD may present with severe adaptive problems, and these problems may become even more serious with development, recommending for early intensive intervention programs* for not only the neuropsychological weaknesses but also the adaptive consequences. As we have stressed in the guidelines presented in Chapter 7, the definition of an intervention program for an individual with NLD must adopt a broad perspective, taking into account not only the neuropsychological deficits and the related intervention but also the areas where the individual meets the most serious adaptive challenges.

• *Research on intervention with NLD is scarce and limited primarily to single cases or small numbers of subjects, whereas a relatively broad series of suggestions is available that can help in identifying some guidelines for intervention.* Guidelines may be useful as a starting point, but science requires appropriate well-designed research. It will not be easy to find resources for the NLD researchers— nor for intervention work within the NLD community—until the clinical category has received recognition.

• *The study of NLD may not only help in understanding the particular group of individuals with NLD but also contribute to the development of knowledge on broader psychological functioning.* For example, we have mentioned in our literature review that research on NLD by Mammarella et al. (2006) offered a new perspective on the differentiation between spatial–simultaneous and spatial–sequential processes.

Suggestions for the Present and Moving Forward

• *Given the absence of the NLD category in the main diagnostic classification systems, a plausible suggestion for clinical diagnosis is to use the available diagnostic categories, stressing, however, the presence of the NLD profile*—for example, "specific LD with (or due to) an NLD profile," "DCD with (or due to) an NLD profile." Although this would be a step forward, it would also create some confusion for practitioners who are not familiar with NLD and would not completely eliminate the problem of access to legislation-mandated services for children with special education needs, to the extent that the NLD profile is often not mentioned and considered. We believe that efforts toward public recognition and specification of the right to be supported within a disability framework are warranted. To our knowledge, Italy is one of the few countries where the definition of provisions for children with special education needs specifically mentions NLD (see Ministero dell'Istruzione . . . , 2013). This inclusive definition has helped in identifying and supporting children with NLD within schools, without the need to also make reference to other diagnostic categories.

• *Until there is formal recognition of NLD, we suggest that interventions for NLD should not be guided by the associated diagnostic label* (e.g., LD) but should be based on the clinical report of the NLD profile. In fact, if the absence of shared criteria forces clinicians to another diagnostic category, greater attention must be devoted to ensure that the intervention is not routinely carried out using the typical procedures adopted for that category. For example, it is well known that many children with dyslexia also have mathematics problems (Andersson & Lyxell, 2007), but it is immediately understandable that the intervention for these children should differ from children who present only with developmental dyscalculia. Similarly, children with NLD and mathematics difficulties should require a different intervention than children with developmental dyscalculia.

• *With the development of knowledge on NLD, it may be expected that–as for other neurodevelopmental disorders–different shared specifications for, and eventually subtypes of, NLD will be described,* with implications for diagnosis and intervention. Previous studies (e.g., Grodzinsky et al., 2010) have already proposed different subtypes of NLD, but we think it is unwise at present to push for subtypes within a category that is still under debate. The criteria we have proposed in Chapter 5 for the diagnosis of NLD (see Criteria C and B, specifying that, respectively, weaknesses should appear in at least one or two of the areas considered) may inherently suggest the individuation of minor differences within the NLD profile, without the need to specify different subtypes. However, we do not exclude the possibility that more well-delineated subtypes can be proposed in the future.

• *The identification of the NLD profile is an example of psychological problems that are poorly compatible with traditional psychiatric approaches, based on taxonomies and the identification of a specific area of weakness,* whereas these problems are more compatible with a dimensional approach that considers a single individual's functioning along different dimensions and the possibility that some weaknesses are grouped in clusters. This is an important point also considered by the DSM-5 (American Psychiatric Association, 2013) and frequently mentioned in the recent literature on psychopathological problems and comorbidity (e.g., Pennington, 2006). We cannot foresee future developments in the field of psychopathology, but we have the impression that a tendency toward recognizing the association between different problems and clinical profiles is gaining popularity, bringing more natural flexibility to a rigid classification system.

In conclusion, we advocate that the absence of an NLD category in the main diagnostic classification systems does not justify the reduction of interest in and efforts on behalf of children with NLD, as these children do exist and often present with problems more serious than those of children with other identified diagnoses. At present it is difficult to expect that public health systems will devote greater attention and more resources to a still-questioned constellation of symptoms. However, parents and teachers who observe the everyday challenges of children with NLD—and the children themselves—are surely deserving of efforts to help maximize resiliency and optimize lifespan outcomes.

References

Achenbach, T. M. (1991). *Child Behavior Checklist/4–18*. Burlington: University of Vermont.

Alloway, T. P., & Archibald, L. (2008). Working memory and learning in children with developmental coordination disorder and specific language impairment. *Journal of Learning Disabilities, 41*(3), 251–262.

Alloway, T. P., Gathercole, S. E., & Pickering, S. J. (2006). Verbal and visuospatial short-term and working memory in children: Are they separable? *Child Development, 77*, 1698–1716.

Alloway, T. P., & Passolunghi, M. C. (2011). The relationship between working memory, IQ, and mathematical skills in children. *Learning and Individual Differences, 21*(1), 133–137.

Al-Yagon, M., Cavendish, W., Cornoldi, C., Fawcett, A. J., Grünke, M., Hung, L. Y., et al. (2013). The proposed changes for DSM-5 for SLD and ADHD: International perspectives—Australia, Germany, Greece, India, Israel, Italy, Spain, Taiwan, United Kingdom, and United States. *Journal of Learning Disabilities, 46*(1), 58–72.

American Psychiatric Association. (1952). *Diagnostic and statistical manual of mental disorders* (1st ed.). Washington, DC: Author.

American Psychiatric Association. (2000). *Diagnostic and statistical manual of mental disorders* (4th ed., text rev.) Washington, DC: Author.

American Psychiatric Association. (2013). *Diagnostic and statistical manual of mental disorders* (5th ed.). Arlington, VA: Author.

Andersson, U., & Lyxell, B. (2007). Working memory deficit in children with mathematical difficulties: A general or specific deficit? *Journal of Experimental Child Psychology, 96*, 197–228.

Antshel, K. M., & Joseph, G. R. (2006). Maternal stress in nonverbal learning disorder: A comparison with reading disorder. *Journal of Learning Disabilities, 39*(3), 194–205.

Antshel, K. M., & Khan, F. M. (2008). Is there an increased familial prevalence of psychopathology in children with nonverbal learning disorders? *Journal of Learning Disabilities, 41*(3), 208–217.

Bachot, J., Gevers, W., Fias, W., & Roeyers, H. (2005). Number sense in children with visuospatial disabilities: Orientation of the mental number line. *Psychology Science, 47,* 172–183.

Baron, I. S. (2004). *Neuropsychological evaluation of the child.* New York: Oxford University Press.

Basso Garcia, R., Mammarella, I. C., Tripodi, D., & Cornoldi, C. (2014). Visuospatial working memory for locations, colours and binding in typically developing children and in children with dyslexia and nonverbal learning disability. *British Journal of Developmental Psychology, 32,* 17–33.

Bauman, M. L., & Kemper, T. L. (2005). Neuroanatomic observations of the brain in autism: A review and future directions. *International Journal of Developmental Neuroscience, 23*(2), 183–187.

Bauminger, N., Edelsztein, H. S., & Morash, J. (2005). Social information processing and emotional understanding in children with LD. *Journal of Learning Disabilities, 38*(1), 45–61.

Beery, K. E., & Buktenica, N. A. (2006). *VMI: Developmental Test of Visual–Motor Integration* (5th ed.). San Antonio, TX: Pearson.

Beery, K. E., Buktenica, N. A., & Beery, N. A. (2010). *Beery–Buktenika developmental test of visual–motor integration, sixth edition.* San Antonio, TX: Pearson Education.

Bender, L. (1946). *Bender Visual Motor Gestalt Test.* New York: American Orthopsychiatric Association.

Bender, W. N., & Golden, L. B. (1990). Subtypes of students with learning disabilities as derived from cognitive, academic, behavioral, and self-concept measures. *Learning Disability Quarterly, 13*(3), 183–194.

Benton, A. L., Sivan, A. B., Hamsher, K. D., Varney, N. R., & Spreen, O. (1994). *Contributions to neuropsychological assessment.* Orlando, FL: Psychological Assessment Resources.

Binet, A., & Simon, T. (1948). The development of the Binet–Simon Scale, 1905–1908. In D. Wayne (Ed.), *Readings in the history of psychology: Century psychology series* (pp. 412–424). East Norwalk, CT: Appleton-Century-Crofts.

Bloom, E., & Heath, N. (2010). Recognition, expression, and understanding facial expression of emotion in adolescents with nonverbal and general learning disabilities. *Journal of Learning Disabilities, 43,* 180–192.

Bölte, S., Holtmann, M., & Poustka, F. (2008). The Social Communication Questionnaire (SCQ) as a screener for autism spectrum disorders: Additional evidence and cross-cultural validity. *Journal of the American Academy of Child and Adolescent Psychiatry, 47,* 719–720.

Bolton, P. F., Carcani-Rathwell, I., Hutton, J., Goode, S., Howlin, P., & Rutter, M. (2011). Epilepsy in autism: Features and correlates. *British Journal of Psychiatry, 198*(4), 289–294.

Bond, L., Butler, H., Thomas, L., Carlin, J., Glover, S., Bowes, G., et al. (2007). Social and school connectedness in early secondary school as predictors of late teenage substance use, mental health, and academic outcomes. *Journal of Adolescent Health, 40*(4), 357.

Bonner, M. J., Hardy, K. K., Willard, V. W., & Gururangan, S. (2009). Additional evidence of a nonverbal learning disability in survivors of pediatric brain tumors. *Children's Health Care, 38*(1), 49–63.

Boone, D. R., & Plante, E. (1993). *Human communication and its disorders.* Englewood Cliffs, NJ: Prentice Hall.

Boshes, B., & Myklebust, H. (1964). General scientific session in conjunction with section on neurology of behavior. *Neurology, 14*(3), 250.

Bowers, L., Huisingh, R., & LoGiudice, C. (2005). *Test of Problem Solving 3: Elementary.* East Moline, IL: LinguiSystems.

Bowers, L., Huisingh, R., & LoGiudice, C. (2008). *Social Language Development Test: Elementary.* East Moline, IL: LinguiSystems.

Bracken, B. A. (1992). *Multidimensional Self Concept Scale.* Austin, TX: PRO-ED.

Breaux, K. C. (2009). *Wechsler Individual Achievement Test–Third Edition.* San Antonio, TX: Pearson.

Broitman, J., & Davis, J. M. (2013). *Treating NVLD in children: Professional collaborations for positive outcomes.* New York: Springer.

Brumback, R. A., & Staton, R. D. (1982). An hypothesis regarding the commonality of right-hemisphere involvement in learning disability, attentional disorder, and childhood major depressive disorder. *Perceptual and Motor Skills, 55*(3, Pt. 2), 1091–1097.

Bull, R., & Scerif, G. (2001). Executive functioning as a predictor of children's mathematics ability: Inhibition, switching, and working memory. *Developmental Neuropsychology, 19*(3), 273–293.

Bunton, L. J., & Fogarty, G. J. (2003). The factor structure of visual imagery and spatial abilities. *Intelligence, 31*, 289–318.

Canetti, E. (1979). *The tongue set free: Remembrance of a European childhood.* New York: Seabury Press.

Cardillo, R., Mammarella, I. C., Basso Garcia, R., & Cornoldi, C. (2016). *Local and global processing in block design tasks in children with dyslexia or nonverbal learning disabilities.* Manuscript submitted for publication.

Carey, M. E., Barakat, L. P., Foley, B., Gyato, K., & Phillips, P. C. (2001). Neuropsychological functioning and social functioning of survivors of pediatric brain tumors: Evidence of nonverbal learning disability. *Child Neuropsychology, 7*(4), 265–272.

Caron, M. J., Mottron, L., Berthiaume, C., & Dawson, M. (2006). Cognitive mechanisms, specificity and neural underpinnings of visuospatial peaks in autism. *Brain, 129*(7), 1789–1802.

Casey, J. E., Rourke, B. P., & Picard, E. M. (1991). Syndrome of nonverbal learning disabilities: Age differences in neuropsychological, academic, and socioemotional functioning. *Development and Psychopathology, 3*, 329–345.

Caviola, S., Toso, C., & Mammarella, I. C. (2011). Impairment of visual working memory in nonverbal learning disability: A treatment case study. *Psicologia Clinica dello Sviluppo, 15*(3), 647–668.

Chandler, S., Charman, T., Baird, G., Simonoff, E., Loucas, T., Meldrum, D., et al. (2007). Validation of the social communication questionnaire in a population cohort of children with autism spectrum disorders. *Journal of the American Academy of Child and Adolescent Psychiatry, 46*(10), 1324–1332.

Chow, D., & Skuy, M. (1999). Simultaneous and successive cognitive processing in children with nonverbal learning disabilities. *School Psychology International, 20*(2), 219–231.

Chronis, A. M., Chacko, A., Fabiano, G. A., Wymbs, B. T., & Pelham Jr., W. E. (2004). Enhancements to the behavioral parent training paradigm for families of children with ADHD: Review and future directions. *Clinical Child and Family Psychology Review, 7*(1), 1–27.

Cianchetti, C., & Sannio Fancello, G. (2001). *SAFA: Scale psichiatriche di autosomministrazione per fanciulli e adolescenti.* Florence, Italy: Giunti O.S.-Organizzazioni Speciali.

Cohen, J. (1988). *Statistical power analysis for the behavioral sciences.* Hillsdale, NJ: Erlbaum.

Cohen, M. (1997). *Children's Memory Scale (CMS).* San Antonio, TX: Psychological Corp.

Colarusso, R., & Hammill, D. (2003). *MVPT-3: Motor-Free Visual Perception Test (MVPT).* Austin, TX: PRO-ED.

Colarusso, R. P., & Hammill, D. D. (1972). *Motor-Free Visual Perceptual Test.* Novato, CA: Academic Therapy.

Collins, A., Brown, J. S., & Newman, S. E. (1989). Cognitive apprenticeship: Teaching the crafts of reading, writing, and mathematics. In L. B. Resnick (Ed.), *Knowing, learning, and instruction: Essays in honor of Robert Glaser* (pp. 453–494). Hillsdale, NJ: Erlbaum.

Connolly, A. J. (2007). *KeyMath 3: Diagnostic assessment.* Bloomington, MN: Pearson.

Cornetti, L. (2015). *Visual perceptual skills in children with nonverbal learning disabilities.* Master's degree dissertation, University of Padua, Italy.

Cornoldi, C., & Cazzola, C. (2003). *AC-MT 11–14: Test di valutazione delle abilità di calcolo e problem solving dagli 11 ai 14 anni.* Trent, Italy: Erickson.

Cornoldi, C., & Colpo, G. (1998). *Prove di lettura MT per la scuola elementare.* Florence, Italy: Giunti O.S.-Organizzazioni Speciali.

Cornoldi, C., dalla Vecchia, R. D., & Tressoldi, P. E. (1995). Visuo-spatial working memory limitations in low visuo-spatial high verbal intelligence children. *Journal of Child Psychology and Psychiatry, 36*(6), 1053–1064.

Cornoldi, C., Ficili, P., Giofrè, D., Mammarella, I. C., & Mirandola, C. (2011). Imaginative representations of two- and three-dimensional matrices in children with nonverbal learning disabilities. *Imagination, Cognition and Personality, 31*(1), 53–62.

Cornoldi, C., Friso, G., Giordano, L., Molin, A., Poli, S., Rigoni, F., et al. (1997). *Abilità visuo-spaziali.* Trent, Italy: Erickson.

Cornoldi, C., & Guglielmo, A. (2001). Children who cannot imagine. *Korean Journal of Thinking and Problem Solving, 11*(2), 99–112.

Cornoldi, C., Lucangeli, D., & Bellina, M. (2012). *AC-MT 6–11: Test di valutazione delle abilità di calcolo e soluzione di problemi.* Trent, Italy: Erickson.

Cornoldi, C., & Mammarella, I. C. (2008). A comparison of backward and forward spatial spans. *Quarterly Journal of Experimental Psychology, 61*(5), 674–682.

Cornoldi, C., Rigoni, F., Tressoldi, P. E., & Vio, C. (1999). Imagery deficits in nonverbal learning disabilities. *Journal of Learning Disabilities, 32*(1), 48–57.

Cornoldi, C., Rigoni, F., Venneri, A., & Vecchi, T. (2000). Passive and active processes in visuo-spatial memory: Double dissociation in developmental learning disabilities. *Brain and Cognition, 43*, 17–20.

Cornoldi, C., & Soresi, S. (1980). *La diagnosi psicologica nelle difficoltà d'apprendimento.* Pordenone, Italy: ERIP.

Cornoldi, C., & Vecchi, T. (2003). *Visuo-spatial working memory and individual differences.* Hove, UK: Psychology Press.

Cornoldi, C., Venneri, A., Marconato, F., Molin, A., & Montinari, C. (2003). A rapid screening measure for the identification of visuospatial learning disability in schools. *Journal of Learning Disabilities, 36*(4), 299–306.

Corsi, P. M. (1972). *Human memory and the medial temporal region of the brain.* Unpublished PhD dissertation, McGill University, Montreal, Quebec, Canada.

Crick, N. R., & Dodge, K. A. (1994). A review and reformulation of social information-processing mechanisms in children's social adjustment. *Psychological Bulletin, 115*(1), 74.

Cruickshank, W. M., & Hallahan, D. (1961). *Perceptual and learning disabilities in children.* Syracuse, NY: Syracuse University Press.

Cutting, L. E., Koth, C. W., & Denckla, M. B. (2000). How children with neurofibromatosis type 1 differ from "typical" learning disabled clinic attenders: Nonverbal learning disabilities revisited. *Developmental Neuropsychology, 17*(1), 29–47.

Davis, J., & Broitman, J. (2007). Nonverbal learning disabilities: Models of proposed subtypes, part II. *The Educational Therapist, 27*(4), 5–10.

Davis, J. M., & Broitman, J. (2011). *Nonverbal learning disabilities in children: Bridging the gap between science and practice.* New York: Springer.

Dehaene, S., Izard, V., Pica, P., & Spelke, E. (2006). Core knowledge of geometry in an Amazonian indigene group. *Science, 311*(5759), 381–384.

Delis, D. C., Kaplan, E., & Kramer, J. H. (2001). *Delis–Kaplan Executive Function System (D-KEFS).* San Antonio, TX: Psychological Corp.

Delis, D. C., Kramer, J. H., Kaplan, E., & Ober, B. A. (1994). *CVLT-C: California Verbal Learning Test.* San Antonio, TX: National Computer System, Pearson.

Della Sala, S., Gray, C., Baddeley, A. D., & Wilson, L. (1997). *Visual Pattern Test.* Bury St. Edmunds, UK: Thames Valley Test Company.

Dimitrovsky, L., Spector, H., Levy-Shiff, R., & Vakil, E. (1998). Interpretation of facial expressions of affect in children with learning disabilities with verbal or nonverbal deficits. *Journal of Learning Disabilities, 31*(3), 286–292.

Drummond, C. R., Ahmad, S. A., & Rourke, B. P. (2005). Rules for the classification of younger children with nonverbal learning disabilities and basic phonological processing disabilities. *Archives of Clinical Neuropsychology, 20*(2), 171–182.

DuPaul, G. J., Reid, R., Anastopoulos, A. D., Lambert, M. C., Watkins, M. W., & Power, T. J. (2016). Parent and teacher ratings of attention-deficit/ hyperactivity disorder symptoms: Factor structure and normative data. *Psychological Assessment, 28*(2), 214–225.

Durand, M. (2005). Is there a fine motor skill deficit in nonverbal learning disabilities? *Educational Child Psychology, 22*, 90–99.

D'Zurilla, T. J., Nezu, A. M., & Maydeu-Olivares, A. (2002). *Social Problem-Solving Inventory–Revised (SPSI-R)*. North Tonawanda, NY: Multi-Health Systems.

Ekman, P., & Friesen, W. V. (1976). *Pictures of facial affect*. Palo Alto, CA: Consulting Psychologists Press.

El-Nokali, N. E., Bachman, H. J., & Votruba-Drzal, E. (2010). Parent involvement and children's academic and social development in elementary school. *Child Development, 81*(3), 988–1005.

Elliot, C. D. (2006). *Differential Ability Scales–Second Edition (DAS–II): Administration and scoring manual*. San Antonio, TX: Psychological Corp.

Etkin, A., Egner, T., & Kalisch, R. (2011). Emotional processing in anterior cingulate and medial prefrontal cortex. *Trends in Cognitive Sciences, 15*(2), 85–93.

Etkin, A., Prater, K. E., Hoeft, F., Menon, V., & Schatzberg, A. F. (2014). Failure of anterior cingulate activation and connectivity with the amygdala during implicit regulation of emotional processing in generalized anxiety disorder. *American Journal of Psychiatry, 167*, 545–554.

Evers, A., Muñiz, J., Bartram, D., Boben, D., Egeland, J., Fernández-Hermida, J. R., et al. (2012). Testing practices in the 21st century. *European Psychologist, 17*, 300–319.

Farrand, P., & Jones, D. (1996). Direction of report in spatial and verbal serial short-term memory. *Quarterly Journal of Experimental Psychology, 49*, 149–158.

Ferrara, R., & Mammarella, I. C. (2013). Il Questionario SVS Bambino. *Psicologia Clinica dello Sviluppo, 2*, 359–368.

Filley, C. M. (2001). *The behavioral neurology of white matter*. New York: Oxford University Press.

Fine, J. G., Musielak, K. A., & Semrud-Clikeman, M. (2014). Smaller splenium in children with nonverbal learning disability compared to controls, high-functioning autism and ADHD. *Child Neuropsychology, 20*(6), 641–661.

Fine, J. G., & Semrud-Clikeman, M. (2010). Nonverbal learning disabilities: Assessment and intervention. In A. S. Davis (Ed.), *Handbook of pediatric neuropsychology* (pp. 721–733). New York: Springer.

Fine, J. G., Semrud-Clikeman, M., Bledsoe, J. C., & Musielak, K. A. (2013). A critical review of the literature on NLD as a developmental disorder. *Child Neuropsychology, 19*(2), 190–223.

Fine, J. G., Semrud-Clikeman, M., Butcher, B., & Walkowiak, J. (2008). Brief report: Attention effect on a measure of social perception. *Journal of Autism and Developmental Disorders, 38*(9), 1797–1802.

Fine, J. G., Semrud-Clikeman, M., & Zhu, D. C. (2009). Gender differences in BOLD activation to face photographs and video vignettes. *Behavioural Brain Research, 201*(1), 137–146.

Fisher, N. J., & Deluca, J. W. (1997). Verbal learning strategies of adolescents and adults with the syndrome of nonverbal learning disabilities. *Child Neuropsychology, 3*(3), 192–198.

Fisher, N. J., Deluca, J. W., & Rourke, B. P. (1997). Wisconsin Card Sorting Test and Halstead Category Test performances of children and adolescents who exhibit the syndrome of nonverbal learning disabilities. *Child Neuropsychology, 3*(1), 61–70.

Fletcher, J. M. (1985). Memory for verbal and nonverbal stimuli in learning disability subgroups: Analysis by selective reminding. *Journal of Experimental Child Psychology, 40*(2), 244–259.

Forrest, B. J. (2004). The utility of math difficulties, internalized psychopathology, and visual–spatial deficits to identify children with the nonverbal learning disability syndrome: Evidence for a visual–spatial disability. *Child Neuropsychology, 10,* 129–146.

Foss, J. M. (1991). Nonverbal learning disabilities and remedial interventions. *Annals of Dyslexia, 41*(1), 128–140.

Frostig, M., & Maslow, P. (1973). *Learning problems in the classroom: Prevention and remediation.* New York: Grune & Stratton.

Fuerst, D. R., Fisk, J. L., & Rourke, B. P. (1990). Psychosocial functioning of learning-disabled children: Relations between WISC Verbal IQ–Performance IQ discrepancies and personality subtypes. *Journal of Consulting and Clinical Psychology, 58*(5), 657.

Fuerst, D. R., & Rourke, B. P. (1993). Psychosocial functioning of children: Relations between personality subtypes and academic achievement. *Journal of Abnormal Child Psychology, 21*(6), 597–607.

Galifret-Granjon, N. (1951). Le problème de l'organisation spatiale dans les dyslexies d'évolution. *Enfance, 4,* 445–479.

Galway, T. M., & Metsala, J. L. (2011). Social cognition and its relation to psychosocial adjustment in children with nonverbal learning disabilities. *Journal of Learning Disabilities, 44*(1), 33–49.

Gau, S. S. F., Lee, C. M., Lai, M. C., Chiu, Y. N., Huang, Y. F., Kao, J. D., et al. (2011). Psychometric properties of the Chinese version of the Social Communication Questionnaire. *Research in Autism Spectrum Disorders, 5*(2), 809–818.

Geary, D. C. (2004). Mathematics and learning disabilities. *Journal of Learning Disabilities, 37*(1), 4–15.

Gerstmann, J. (1940). Syndrome of finger agnosia, disorientation for right and left, agraphia and acalculia. *Archives of Neurology and Psychiatry, 44,* 398–408.

Gilliam, J. (2013). *Gilliam Autism Rating Scale–Third Edition (GARS-3).* Houston: PRO-ED.

Gioia, G. A., Isquith, P. K., Guy, S. C., & Kenworthy, L. (2000). *Behavior Rating Inventory of Executive Function (BRIEF).* Odessa, FL: Psychological Assessment Resources.

Goldberg, E., & Costa, L. D. (1981). Hemisphere differences in the acquisition and use of descriptive systems. *Brain and Language, 14*(1), 144–173.

Goldberg, E., Vaughan, H. G., & Gerstman, L. J. (1978). Nonverbal descriptive systems and hemispheric asymmetry: Shape versus texture discrimination. *Brain and Language, 5*(2), 249–257.

Goldstein, S., & Naglieri, J. (2010). *Autism Spectrum Rating Scales (ASRS)*. Toronto: Multi-Health Systems.

Goodwin, M. H. (1999). Participation. *Journal of Linguistic Anthropology, 9*(1/2), 177–180.

Grabner, R. H., Ansari, D., Koschutnig, K., Reishofer, G., Ebner, F., & Neuper, C. (2009). To retrieve or to calculate?: Left angular gyrus mediates the retrieval of arithmetic facts during problem solving. *Neuropsychologia, 47*(2), 604–608.

Grahn, J. A., Parkinson, J. A., & Owen, A. M. (2008). The cognitive functions of the caudate nucleus. *Progress in Neurobiology, 86*(3), 141–155.

Grodzinsky, G. M., Forbes, P. W., & Bernstein J. H. (2010). A practice-based approach to group identification in nonverbal learning disorders. *Child Neuropsychology, 16*, 433–460.

Groen, W., Teluj, M., Buitelaar, J., & Tendolkar, I. (2010). Amygdala and hippocampus enlargement during adolescence in autism. *Journal of the American Academy of Child and Adolescent Psychiatry, 49*, 552–560.

Grossman, J. B., Klin, A., Carter, A. S., & Volkmar, F. R. (2000). Verbal bias in recognition of facial emotions in children with Asperger syndrome. *Journal of Child Psychology and Psychiatry, 41*(3), 369–379.

Gross-Tsur, V., Shalev, R. S., Manor, O., & Amil, N. (1995). Developmental right hemisphere syndrome: Clinical spectrum of the nonverbal learning disability. *Journal of Learning Disabilities, 28*, 80–86.

Grunau, R. E., Whitfield, M. F., & Davis, C. (2002). Pattern of learning disabilities in children with extremely low birth weight and broadly average intelligence. *Archives of Pediatrics and Adolescent Medicine, 156*(6), 615–620.

Guli, L. A., Semrud-Clikeman, M., Lerner, M. D., & Britton, N. (2013). Social Competence Intervention Program (SCIP): A pilot study of a creative drama program for youth with social difficulties. *Arts in Psychotherapy, 40*(1), 37–44.

Guli, L. A., Wilkinson, A., & Semrud-Clikeman, M. (2008). *Social competence intervention program*. Champaign, IL: Research Press.

Hammill, D. D. (1990). On defining learning disabilities: An emerging consensus. *Journal of Learning Disabilities, 23*, 74–84.

Happé, F. (1999). Autism: Cognitive deficit or cognitive style? *Trends in Cognitive Science, 3*, 216–222.

Harnadek, M. C., & Rourke, B. P. (1994). Principal identifying features of the syndrome of nonverbal learning disabilities in children. *Journal of Learning Disabilities, 27*(3), 144–154.

Hassiotis, A. (1997). Parents of young persons with learning disability: An application of the Family Adaptability and Cohesion Scale (FACES II). *British Journal of Developmental Disabilities, 43*, 36–42.

Hécaen, H., Angelergues, R., & Houillier, S. (1961). Les variétés cliniques des acalculies au cours des lésions rétro-rolandiques: Approche statistique du problème. *Revue Neurologique, 105,* 85–103.

Henderson, S. E., Sugden, D. A., & Barnett, A. L. (2007). *Movement Assessment Battery for Children–2 (Movement ABC-2): Examiner's manual.* London: Harcourt Assessment.

Hendriksen, J. G. M., Keulers, E. H. H., Feron, F. J. M., Wassenberg, R., Jolles, J., & Vles, J. S. H. (2007). Subtypes of learning disabilities: Neuropsychological and behavioral functioning of 495 children referred for multidisciplinary assessment. *European Child Adolescence and Psychiatry, 16,* 517–524.

Hong, D. S., Dunkin, B., & Reiss, A. L. (2011). Psychosocial functioning and social cognitive processing in girls with Turner syndrome. *Journal of Developmental and Behavioral Pediatrics, 32*(7), 512.

Howard, K. A., & Tryon, G. S. (2002). Depressive symptoms in and type of classroom placement for adolescents with LD. *Journal of Learning Disabilities, 35*(2), 185–190.

Hubbard, E. M., Piazza, M., Pinel, P., & Dehaene, S. (2005). Interactions between number and space in parietal cortex. *Nature Reviews Neuroscience, 6*(6), 435–448.

Humphries, T., Cardy, J. O., Worling, D. E., & Peets, K. (2004). Narrative comprehension and retelling abilities of children with nonverbal learning disabilities. *Brain and Cognition, 56*(1), 77–88.

Individuals with Disabilities Education Act, Pub. L. No. 91-230, 84 Stat. 191 (1970).

Inglis, J., & Lawson, J. S. (1987). Reanalysis of a meta-analysis of the validity of the Wechsler Scales in the diagnosis of learning disability. *Learning Disability Quarterly, 10*(3), 198–202.

Iuculano, T., Tang, J., Hall, C. W., & Butterworth, B. (2008). Core information processing deficits in developmental dyscalculia and low numeracy. *Developmental Science, 11*(5), 669–680.

Jastak, J. F., & Jastak, S. R. (1965). *Wide Range Achievement Test: Manual.* Wilmington, DE: Guidance Associates.

Jastak, S. (1984). *WRAT-R: Wide Range Achievement Test.* Chicago: Jastak Associates.

Johnson, D., & Myklebust, H. (1967). *Learning disabilities: Educational principles and practices.* New York: Grune & Stratton.

Johnson-Laird, P. N. (1983). *Mental models: Towards a cognitive science of language, inference, and consciousness (No. 6).* Cambridge, MA: Harvard University Press.

Jones, D., Farrand, P., Stuart, G., & Morris, N. (1995). Functional equivalence of verbal and spatial information in serial short-term memory. *Journal of Experimental Psychology: Learning, Memory, and Cognition, 21*(4), 1008.

Jordan, D. W., & Métais, J. L. (1997). Social skilling through cooperative learning. *Educational Research, 39*(1), 3–21.

Karmiloff-Smith, A. (2010). Neuroimaging of the developing brain: Taking "developing" seriously. *Human Brain Mapping, 31*(6), 934–941.

Kaufman, A. S., & Kaufman, N. L. (1983). *K-ABC: Kaufman Assessment Battery for Children: Interpretive manual.* Circle Pines, MN: American Guidance Service.

Kaufman, A. S., & Kaufman, N. L. (2004). *Kaufman Assessment Battery for Children* (2nd ed.). Circle Pines, MN: American Guidance Service.

Kazdin, A. E., Stolar, M. J., & Marciano, P. L. (1995). Risk factors for dropping out of treatment among white and black families. *Journal of Family Psychology, 9*(4), 402.

Kazdin, A. E., & Wassell, G. (2000). Therapeutic changes in children, parents, and families resulting from treatment of children with conduct problems. *Journal of the American Academy of Child and Adolescent Psychiatry, 39*(4), 414–420.

Keith, T. Z., Fine, J. G., Taub, G. E., Reynolds, M. R., & Kranzler, J. H. (2006). Higher order, multisample, confirmatory factor analysis of the Wechsler Intelligence Scale for Children—Fourth Edition: What does it measure? *School Psychology Review, 35*(1), 108–127.

Kephart, N. C. (1960). *The slow learner in the classroom.* Columbus, OH: Merrill.

Kirk, S. A., & Kirk, W. D. (1971). *Psycho-linguistic learning disabilities: Diagnosis and remediation.* Urbana: University of Illinois Press.

Klin, A., Jones, W., Schultz, R., Volkmar, F., & Cohen, D. (2002). Visual fixation patterns during viewing of naturalistic social situations as predictors of social competence in individuals with autism. *Archives of General Psychiatry, 59*(9), 809–816.

Klin, A., Volkmar, F. R., Sparrow, S. S., Cicchetti, D. V., & Rourke, B. P. (1995). Validity and neuropsychological characterization of Asperger syndrome: Convergence with nonverbal learning disabilities syndrome. *Journal of Child Psychology and Psychiatry, 36*(7), 1127–1140.

Kløve, H. (1963). *Grooved pegboard.* Lafayette, IN: Lafayette Instruments.

Kodituwakku, P. W. (2007). Defining the behavioral phenotype in children with fetal alcohol spectrum disorders: A review. *Neuroscience and Biobehavioral Reviews, 31*(2), 192–201.

Koffka, K. (2013). *Principles of Gestalt psychology* (Vol. 44). London: Routledge.

Koppitz, E. M. (1975). Bender Gestalt Test, Visual Aural Digit Span Test and reading achievement. *Journal of Learning Disabilities, 8*(3), 154–158.

Korkman, M., Kirk, U., & Kemp, S. (2007). *NEPSY-II.* San Antonio, TX: Pearson.

Kovacs, M. (2010). *Children's Depression Inventory 2 (CDI 2).* Pittsburgh: University of Pittsburgh School of Medicine.

Krug, D. A., & Arick, J. R. (2003). *Krug Asperger Disorder Index (KADI).* Austin, TX: PRO-ED.

Kyttälä, M. (2008). Visuospatial working memory in adolescents with poor performance in mathematics: Variation depending on reading skills. *Educational Psychology, 28*(3), 273–289.

Lajiness-O'Neill, R., Beaulieu, I., Asamoah, A., Titus, J. B., Bawle, E., Ahmad, S., et al. (2006). The neuropsychological phenotype of velocardiofacial syndrome (VCFS): Relationship to psychopathology. *Archives of Clinical Neuropsychology, 21*(2), 175–184.

Landa, R., Klin, A., & Volkmar, F. (2000). Social language use in Asperger syndrome and high-functioning autism. In A. Klin, F. R. Volkmar, & S. S. Sparrow (Eds.), *Asperger syndrome* (pp. 125–155). New York: Guilford Press.

Landerl, K., Fussenegger, B., Moll, K., & Willburger, E. (2009). Dyslexia and dyscalculia: Two learning disorders with different cognitive profiles. *Journal of Experimental Child Psychology, 103*(3), 309–324.

Larson, E. B., Kirschner, K., Bode, R., Heinemann, A., & Goodman, R. (2005). Construct and predictive validity of the Repeatable Battery for the Assessment of Neuropsychological Status in the evaluation of stroke patients. *Journal of Clinical and Experimental Neuropsychology, 27*(1), 16–32.

Lavoie, R. (1994). *Social competence and the child with learning disabilities.* Washington, DC: WETA-TV. Available at *www.ldonline.org.*

Lawson, J. S., & Inglis, J. (1985). Learning disabilities and intelligence test results: A model based on a principal components analysis of the WISC-R. *British Journal of Psychology, 76*(1), 35–48.

LeCouteur, A., Lord, C., & Rutter, M. (2003). *The Autism Diagnostic Interview–Revised (ADI-R).* Los Angeles: Western Psychological Services.

Lepach, A. C., & Petermann, F. (2011). Nonverbal and verbal learning: A comparative study of children and adolescents with 22q11 deletion syndrome, non-syndromal nonverbal learning disorder and memory disorder. *Neurocase, 17,* 480–490.

Lerner, M. D., Mikami, A. Y., & Levine, K. (2011). Socio-dramatic affective-relational intervention for adolescents with Asperger syndrome: Pilot study. *Autism, 15*(1), 21–42.

Levin, L., & Langton, M. (2007). *The verbal math lesson level 1: Step-by-step math without pencil or paper.* San Ramon, CA: Mountcastle Company.

Lezak, M. D. (1976). *Neuropsychological assessment.* New York: Oxford University Press.

Lezak, M. D., Howicson, D. B., & Loring, D. W. (2004). *Neuropsychological assessment* (4th ed.). New York: Oxford University Press.

Liddell, G. A., & Rasmussen, C. (2005). Memory profile of children with nonverbal learning disability. *Learning Disabilities Research and Practice, 20*(3), 137–141.

Linnenbrink, E. A. (2006). Emotion research in education: Theoretical and methodological perspectives on the integration of affect, motivation, and cognition. *Educational Psychology Review, 18*(4), 307–314.

Lipman, E. L., Offord, D. R., Dooley, M. D., & Boyle, M. H. (2002). Children's outcomes in differing types of single-parent families. In J. D. Willms (Ed.), *Vulnerable children* (pp. 229–242). Edmonton: University of Alberta Press.

Litt, J., Taylor, H. G., Klein, N., & Hack, M. (2005). Learning disabilities in children with very low birthweight: Prevalence, neuropsychological correlates, and educational interventions. *Journal of Learning Disabilities, 38*(2), 130–141.

Little, L. (2002). Middle-class mothers' perceptions of peer and sibling victimization among children with Asperger's syndrome and nonverbal learning disorders. *Issues in Comprehensive Pediatric Nursing, 25*(1), 43–57.

Little, S. S. (1993). Nonverbal learning disabilities and socioemotional functioning: A review of recent literature. *Journal of Learning Disabilities, 26*(10), 653–665.

Logie, R. H. (1995). *Visuo-spatial memory*. Hove, UK: Erlbaum.

Lopez, C., Tchanturia, K., Stahl, D., & Treasure, J. (2008). Central coherence in eating disorders: A systematic review. *Psychological Medicine, 38*(10), 1393–1404.

Maag, J. W., & Reid, R. (2006). Depression among students with learning disabilities assessing the risk. *Journal of Learning Disabilities, 39*(1), 3–10.

Mabbott, D. J., & Bisanz, J. (2008). Computational skills, working memory, and conceptual knowledge in older children with mathematics learning disabilities. *Journal of Learning Disabilities, 41*(1), 15–28.

Magill-Evans, J., Koning, C., Cameron-Sadava, A., & Manyk, K. (1995). The Child and Adolescent Social Perception Measure. *Journal of Nonverbal Behavior, 19*, 151–169.

Magill-Evans, J., Koning, C., Cameron-Sadava, A., & Manyk, K. (1996). *Manual for the Child and Adolescent Social Perception Measure*. Unpublished manuscript.

Mamen, M. (2006). *Nonverbal learning disabilities and their clinical subtypes: A handbook for parents and professionals–new edition*. Ottawa: Centrepointe Professional Services.

Mammarella, I. C., Bomba, M., Caviola, S., Broggi, F., Neri, F., Lucangeli, D., et al. (2013a). Mathematical difficulties in nonverbal learning disability or co-morbid dyscalculia and dyslexia. *Developmental Neuropsychology, 38*(6), 418–432.

Mammarella, I. C., Coltri, S., Lucangeli, D., & Cornoldi, C. (2009a). Impairment of simultaneous–spatial working memory in nonverbal (visuospatial) learning disability: A treatment case study. *Neuropsychological Rehabilitation, 19*(5), 761–780.

Mammarella, I. C., & Cornoldi, C. (2005a). Difficulties in the control of irrelevant visuospatial information in children with visuospatial learning disabilities. *Acta Psychologica, 118*, 211–228.

Mammarella, I. C., & Cornoldi, C. (2005b). Sequence and space: The critical role of a backward spatial span in the working memory deficit of visuospatial learning disabled children. *Cognitive Neuropsychology, 22*, 1055–1068.

Mammarella, I. C., & Cornoldi, C. (2014). An analysis of the criteria used to diagnose children with nonverbal learning disability (NLD). *Child Neuropsychology, 20*(3), 255–280.

Mammarella, I. C., Cornoldi, C., Pazzaglia, F., Toso, C., Grimoldi, M., & Vio, C. (2006). Evidence for a double dissociation between spatial–simultaneous and spatial–sequential working memory in visuospatial (nonverbal) learning disabled children. *Brain and Cognition, 62*, 58–67.

Mammarella, I. C., Giofrè, D., Ferrara, R., & Cornoldi, C. (2013b). Intuitive geometry and visuospatial working memory in children showing symptoms of nonverbal learning disabilities. *Child Neuropsychology, 19*(3), 235–249.

Mammarella, I. C., & Lipparini, S. (2015). Un intervento sulla comprensione del testo e sul metodo di studio in un caso di disturbo dell'apprendimento non verbale. *Psicologia Clinica dello Sviluppo, 19*(1), 165–176.

Mammarella, I. C., Lucangeli, D., & Cornoldi, C. (2010a). Spatial working memory and arithmetic deficits in children with nonverbal learning difficulties. *Journal of Learning Disabilities, 43*, 455–468.

Mammarella, I. C., Meneghetti, C., Pazzaglia, F., & Cornoldi, C. (2015). Memory and comprehension deficits in spatial descriptions in children with nonverbal and reading disabilities. *Frontiers in Developmental Psychology, 5*, 1534.

Mammarella, I. C., Meneghetti, C., Pazzaglia. F., Gitti, F., Gomez, C., & Cornoldi, C. (2009b). Representation of survey and route spatial descriptions in children with nonverbal (visuospatial) learning disabilities. *Brain and Cognition, 71*, 173–179.

Mammarella, I. C., & Pazzaglia, F. (2010). Visual perception and memory impairments in children at risk of nonverbal learning disabilities. *Child Neuropsychology, 16*(6), 564–576.

Mammarella, I. C., Pazzaglia, F., & Cornoldi, C. (2008a). Evidence for different components in children's visuospatial working memory. *British Journal of Developmental Psychology, 26*(3), 337–355.

Mammarella, I. C., Toso, C., & Caviola, S. (2010b). *Memoria di lavoro visuospaziale. Attività per il recupero e il potenziamento* [Visuospatial working memory: Training activities]. Trent, Italy: Erickson.

Mammarella, I. C., Toso, C., Pazzaglia, F., & Cornoldi, C. (2008b). *BVS-Corsi. Batteria per la valutazione della memoria visiva e spaziale.* Trent, Italy: Erickson.

March, J. S. (2012). *Multidimensional Anxiety Scale for Children–Second Edition.* North Tonowanda, NY: Multi-Health Systems.

Margalit, M., Raviv, A., & Ankonina, D. B. (1992). Coping and coherence among parents with disabled children. *Journal of Clinical Child and Adolescent Psychology, 21*(3), 202–209.

Margalit, M., & Shulman, S. (1986). Autonomy perceptions and anxiety expressions of learning disabled adolescents. *Journal of Learning Disabilities, 19*(5), 291–293.

Marsh, H. W., & Martin, A. J. (2011). Academic self-concept and academic achievement: Relations and causal ordering. *British Journal of Educational Psychology, 81*(1), 59–77.

Matson, J. L., Matson, M. L., & Rivet, T. T. (2007). Social-skills treatments for children with autism spectrum disorders: An overview. *Behavior Modification, 31*(5), 682–707.

Matte, R. R., & Bolaski, J. A. (1998). Nonverbal learning disabilities: An overview. *Intervention in School and Clinic, 34*(1), 39–42.

Mattson, A. J., Sheer, D. E., & Fletcher, J. M. (1992). Electrophysiological evidence of lateralized disturbances in children with learning disabilities. *Journal of Clinical and Experimental Neuropsychology, 14*(5), 707–716.

Mazzocco, M. M. (2001). Math learning disability and math LD subtypes: Evidence from studies of Turner syndrome, fragile X syndrome, and neurofibromatosis type 1. *Journal of Learning Disabilities, 34*(6), 520–533.

Mazzocco, M. M., & Myers, G. F. (2003). Complexities in identifying and defining mathematics learning disability in the primary school-age years. *Annals of Dyslexia, 53*(1), 218–253.

McCarney, D., & Greenberg, L. M. (1990). *Test of Variables of Attention (TOVA).* Minneapolis, MN: Attention Technology.

McDougall, J., DeWitt, D. J., King, G., Miller, T., & Killip, S. (2004). High school-aged youths' attitudes toward their peers with disabilities: The role of school and student interpersonal factors. *International Journal of Disability, Development and Education, 51,* 287–313.

McDowell, A. D., Saylor, C. F., Taylor, M. J., Boyce, G. C., & Stokes, S. J. (1995). Ethnicity and parenting stress change during early intervention. *Early Child Development and Care, 111*(1), 131–140.

McGinnis, E., & Goldstein, A. P. (1997). *Skillstreaming the elementary school child: New strategies and perspectives for teaching prosocial skills.* Champaign, IL: Research Press.

McGrew, K. S. (2009). CHC theory and the human cognitive abilities project: Standing on the shoulders of the giants of psychometric intelligence research. *Intelligence, 37,* 1–10.

McLean, J. F., & Hitch, G. J. (1999). Working memory impairments in children with specific arithmetic learning difficulties. *Journal of Experimental Child Psychology, 74*(3), 240–260.

Meltzer, L. (2007). *Executive function in education: From theory to practice.* New York: Guilford Press.

Meyers, J. E., & Meyers, K. R. (1995). *Rey Complex Figure and Recognition Trial: Professional manual.* Odessa, FL: Psychological Assessment Resources.

Meyers, J. E., & Meyers, K. R. (1996). *Rey Complex Figure Test and Recognition Trial: Supplemental norms for children and adults.* Odessa, FL: Psychological Assessment Resources.

Ministero dell'Instruzione, della'Università e della Ricerca. (2013). *Circolare Ministeriale n. 8 del 06.03.2013 con le Indicazioni Operative della Direttiva Ministeriale del 27.12.2012 "Strumenti d'intervento per alunni con bisogni educativi speciali e organizzazione territoriale per l'inclusione scolastica."* Rome: Author.

Mirandola, C., Losito, N., Ghetti, S., & Cornoldi, C. (2014). Emotional false memories in children with learning disabilities. *Research in Developmental Disabilities, 35,* 261–268.

Moes, D., Koegel, R. L., Schreibman, L., & Loos, L. M. (1992). Stress profiles for mothers and fathers of children with autism. *Psychological Reports, 71*(3 Pt. 2), 1272–1274.

Montessori, M. (1934). *Psicogeométria.* Barcelona, Spain: Araluce.

Murphy, M. M., Mazzocco, M. M., Hanich, L. B., & Early, M. C. (2007). Cognitive characteristics of children with mathematics learning disability (MLD) vary as a function of the cutoff criterion used to define MLD. *Journal of Learning Disabilities, 40*(5), 458–478.

Myklebust, H. R. (1975). Nonverbal learning disabilities: Assessment and interventions. In H. R. Myklebust (Ed.), *Progress in learning disabilities* (Vol. 3, pp. 85–121). New York: Grune & Stratton.

Nichelli, P., & Venneri, A. (1995). Right hemisphere developmental learning disability: A case study. *Neurocase, 1*(2), 173–177.

Nowicki, S., Jr., & Duke, M. P. (1994). Individual differences in the nonverbal communication of affect: The Diagnostic Analysis of Nonverbal Accuracy Scale. *Journal of Nonverbal Behavior, 18*(1), 9–35.

Orton, S. T. (1937). *Reading, writing and speech problems in children.* New York: Norton.

Osmon, D. C., Smerz, J. M., Braun, M. M., & Plambeck, E. (2006). Processing abilities associated with math skills in adult learning disability. *Journal of Clinical and Experimental Neuropsychology, 28,* 84–95.

Osterrieth, P. A. (1944). Le test de copie d'une figure complèxe. *Archives de Psychologie, 30,* 206–356.

Ozols, E. J., & Rourke, B. P. (1991). Characteristics of young learning-disabled children classified according to patterns of academic achievement: Validity studies. In B. P. Rourke (Ed.), *Neuropsychological validation of learning disability subtypes* (pp. 97–123). New York: Guilford Press.

Ozonoff, S., & Rogers, S. J. (2003). From Kanner to the millennium. In S. Ozonoff, S. J. Rogers, & R. L. Hendren (Eds.), *Autism spectrum disorders: A research review for practitioners* (pp. 3–33). Arlington, VA: American Psychiatric Publishing.

Pagel, J. (1901). *Biographisches Lexikon her-vorragender Arzte des neunzehnten Jahrhun-derts* [Biographical dictionary of excellent doctors from the nineteenth century]. Berlin: Urban & Schwarzenberg.

Pagulayan, K. F., Busch, R. M., Medina, K. L., Bartok, J. A., & Krikorian, R. (2006). Developmental normative data for the Corsi Block-Tapping Task. *Journal of Clinical and Experimental Neuropsychology, 28,* 1043–1052.

Palombo, J. (2006). *Nonverbal learning disabilities: A clinical perspective.* New York: Norton.

Passolunghi, M. C., & Mammarella, I. C. (2010). Spatial and visual working memory ability in children with difficulties in arithmetic word problem solving. *European Journal of Cognitive Psychology, 22*(6), 944–963.

Passolunghi, M. C., & Siegel, L. S. (2001). Short-term memory, working memory, and inhibitory control in children with difficulties in arithmetic problem solving. *Journal of Experimental Child Psychology, 80*(1), 44–57.

Passolunghi, M. C., & Siegel, L. S. (2004). Working memory and access to numerical information in children with disability in mathematics. *Journal of Experimental Child Psychology, 88*(4), 348–367.

Pazzaglia, F., & Cornoldi, C. (1999). The role of distinct components of visuo–spatial working memory in the processing of texts. *Memory, 7*(1), 19–41.

Pedroni, B., Molin, A., & Cornoldi, C. (2007). Difficoltà di apprendimento visuospaziali: Il questionario SVS per uno screening nelle scuole secondarie inferiori. *Difficoltà di Apprendimento, 13,* 207–224.

Pelletier, P. M., Ahmad, S. A., & Rourke, B. P. (2001). Classification rules for basic phonological processing disabilities and nonverbal learning disabilities: Formulation and external validity. *Child Neuropsychology, 7,* 84–98.

Pennington, B. F. (1991). Right hemisphere learning disorders. In *Diagnosing learning disorders: A neuropsychological framework* (pp. 111–134). New York: Guilford Press.

Pennington, B. F. (2006). From single to multiple deficit models of developmental disorders. *Cognition, 101*, 385–413.

Petti, V. L., Voelker, S. L., Shore, D. L., & Hayman-Abello, S. E. (2003). Perception of nonverbal emotion cues by children with nonverbal learning disabilities. *Journal of Developmental and Physical Disabilities, 15*(1), 23–36.

Puig-Antich, J., & Chambers, W. (1978). *The Schedule for Affective Disorders and Schizophrenia for School-Age Children (Kiddie-SADS).* New York: New York State Psychiatric Institute.

Ralston, M. B., Fuerst, D. R., & Rourke, B. P. (2003). Comparison of the psychosocial typology of children with below average IQ to that of children with learning disabilities. *Journal of Clinical and Experimental Neuropsychology, 25*(2), 255–273.

Raver, C. C., Jones, S. M., Li-Grining, C., Zhai, F., Bub, K., & Pressler, E. (2011). CSRP's impact on low-income preschoolers' preacademic skills: Self-regulation as a mediating mechanism. *Child Development, 82*(1), 362–378.

Reddon, J. R., Gill, D. M., Gauk, S. E., & Maerz, M. D. (1988). Purdue Pegboard: Test–retest estimates. *Perceptual and Motor Skills, 66*(2), 503–506.

Reitan, R. M., & Wolfson, D. (1985). *The Halstead–Reitan Neuropsychological Test Battery: Theory and clinical interpretation.* Tucson, AZ: Neuropsychology Press.

Rey, A. (1941). L'examen psychologique dans les cas d'encephalopathie traumatique. *Archives de Psychologie, 28*, 286–340.

Rey, A. (1967). *Reattivo della figura complessa.* Florence, Italy: Giunti O.S.-Organizzazioni Speciali.

Reynolds, C. R., & Kamphaus, R. W. (2004). *BASC-2: Behavior Assessment System for Children, Second Edition manual.* Circle Pines, MN: American Guidance Service.

Reynolds, C. R., & Richmond, B. O. (2008). *Revised Children's Manifest Anxiety Scale, Second Edition (RCMAS-2): Manual.* Los Angeles: Western Psychological Services.

Reynolds, C. R., & Voress, J. (2007). *Test of Memory and Learning (TOMAL-2).* Austin, TX: Pro-Ed.

Richardson, G. P. (1999). *Feedback thought in social science and systems theory.* Cambridge, MA: Pegasus Communications.

Rigoni, F., Cornoldi, C., & Alcetti, A. (1997). Difficoltà nella comprensione e rappresentazione di descrizioni visuospaziali in bambini con disturbi non-verbali dell'apprendimento. *Psicologia Clinica dello Sviluppo, 1*(2), 189–218.

Ris, M. D., Ammerman, R. T., Waller, N., Walz, N., Oppenheimer, S., Brown, T., et al. (2007). Taxonicity of nonverbal learning disabilities in spina bifida. *Journal of the International Neuropsychological Society, 13*(1), 50–58.

Ris, M. D., & Nortz, M. (2008). Nonverbal learning disorder. In J. E. Morgan & J. H. Ricker (Eds.), *Textbook of clinical neuropsychology* (pp. 346–359). East Sussex, UK: Taylor & Francis.

Roid, G. H. (2003). *Stanford–Binet intelligence scales (SB5)*. Rolling Meadows, IL: Riverside.

Rourke, B. P. (1985). *Neuropsychology of learning disabilities: Essentials of subtype analysis*. New York: Guilford Press.

Rourke, B. P. (1987). Syndrome of nonverbal learning disabilities: The final common pathway of white-matter disease/dysfunction? *The Clinical Neuropsychologist, 1*(3), 209–234.

Rourke, B. P. (1989). *Nonverbal learning disabilities: The syndrome and the model*. New York: Guilford Press.

Rourke, B. P. (1995). *Syndrome of nonverbal learning disabilities: Neurodevelopmental manifestations*. New York: Guilford Press.

Rourke, B. P. (2000). Neuropsychological and psychosocial subtyping: A review of investigations within the University of Windsor laboratory. *Canadian Psychology, 41*(1), 34–51.

Rourke, B. P., & Finlayson, A. J. (1978). Neuropsychological significance of variations in patterns of academic performance: Verbal and visuo–spatial abilities. *Journal of Abnormal Child Psychology, 6*, 121–133.

Rourke, B. P., & Finlayson, M. A. (1975). Neuropsychological significance of variations in patterns of performance on the Trail Making Test for older children with learning disabilities. *Journal of Abnormal Psychology, 84*(4), 412.

Rourke, B. P., & Fuerst, D. R. (1992). Psychosocial dimensions of learning disability subtypes: Neuropsychological studies in the Windsor Laboratory. *School Psychology Review, 21*, 360–373.

Rourke, B. P., & Gates, R. D. (1981). Neuropsychological research and school psychology. In G. Hynd & J. E. Obrzut (Eds.), *Neuropsychological assessment and the school-age child: Issues and procedures* (pp. 3–25). New York: Grune & Stratton.

Rourke, B. P., Rourke, S., & van der Vlugt, H. (2002). *Practice of child-clinical neuropsychology: An introduction*. Boca Raton, FL: CRC Press.

Rourke, B. P., & Strang, J. D. (1978). Neuropsychological significance of variations in patterns of academic performance: Motor, psychomotor, and tactile–perceptual abilities. *Journal of Pediatric Psychology, 3*(2), 62–66.

Rourke, B. P., & Tsatsanis, K. D. (1996). Syndrome of nonverbal learning disabilities: Psycholinguistic assets and deficits. *Topics in Language Disorders, 16*(2), 30–44.

Rourke, B. P., Young, G. C., & Leenaars, A. A. (1989). A childhood learning disability that predisposes those afflicted to adolescent and adult depression and suicide risk. *Journal of Learning Disabilities, 22*(3), 169–175.

Rueger, S. Y., Malecki, C. K., & Demaray, M. K. (2010). Relationship between multiple sources of perceived social support and psychological and academic adjustment in early adolescence: Comparisons across gender. *Journal of Youth and Adolescence, 39*(1), 47–61.

Rutter, M., DiLavore, P. C., Risi, S., Gotham, K., & Bishop, S. L. (2012). *Autism Diagnostic Observation Schedule: ADOS-2*. Los Angeles: Western Psychological Services.

Rutter, M., LeCouteur, A., & Lord, C. (2003). *Autism Diagnostic Interview–Revised manual*. Los Angeles: Western Psychological Services.

Ryburn, B., Anderson, V., & Wales, R. (2009). Asperger syndrome: How does it relate to non-verbal learning disability? *Journal of Neuropsychology, 3*(1), 107–123.

Sandson, T. A., Bachna, K. J., & Morin, M. D. (2000). Right hemisphere dysfunction in ADHD visual hemispatial inattention and clinical subtype. *Journal of Learning Disabilities, 33*(1), 83–90.

Schiff, R., Bauminger, N., & Toledo, I. (2009). Analogical problem solving in children with verbal and nonverbal learning disabilities. *Journal of Learning Disabilities, 42*, 3–13.

Schmidt, S. F. (2011). *Life of Fred elementary series*. Reno, NV: Polka Dot.

Schoemaker, M. M. (2008). *MOQ-T Motor Observation Questionnaire for Teachers: Manual*. Groningen, The Netherlands: Center for Human Movement Sciences, University Medical Center Groningen.

Schopler, E., Van Bourgondien, M. E., Wellman, G. J., & Love, S. R. (2010). *CARS 2: Childhood Autism Rating Scale*. Los Angeles: Western Psychological Services.

Semrud-Clikeman, M., & Fine, J. (2011). Presence of cysts on magnetic resonance images (MRIs) in children with Asperger disorder and nonverbal learning disabilities. *Journal of Child Neurology, 26*(4), 471–475.

Semrud-Clikeman, M., Fine, J. G., & Bledsoe, J. (2014). Comparison among children with children with autism spectrum disorder, nonverbal learning disorder and typically developing children on measures of executive functioning. *Journal of Autism and Developmental Disorders, 44*(2), 331–342.

Semrud-Clikeman, M., Fine, J. G., Bledsoe, J., & Zhu, D. C. (2013). Magnetic resonance imaging volumetric findings in children with Asperger syndrome, nonverbal learning disability, or healthy controls. *Journal of Clinical and Experimental Neuropsychology, 35*(5), 540–550.

Semrud-Clikeman, M., & Glass, K. (2008). Comprehension of humor in children with nonverbal learning disabilities, reading disabilities, and without learning disabilities. *Annals of Dyslexia, 58*(2), 163–180.

Semrud-Clikeman, M., & Hynd, G. W. (1990). Right hemisphere dysfunction in nonverbal learning disabilities: Social, academic, and adaptive functioning in adults and children. *Psychological Bulletin, 107*(2), 196.

Semrud-Clikeman, M., Walkowiak, J., Wilkinson, A., & Christopher, G. (2010a). Neuropsychological differences among children with Asperger syndrome, nonverbal learning disabilities, attention deficit disorder, and controls. *Developmental Neuropsychology, 35*, 582–600.

Semrud-Clikeman, M., Walkowiak, J., Wilkinson, A., & Portman Minne, E. (2010b). Direct and indirect measures of social perception, behavior, and emotional functioning in children with Asperger's disorder, nonverbal learning disability, or ADHD. *Journal of Abnormal Child Psychology, 38*, 509–519.

Shaw, P., Gilliam, M., Liverpool, M., Weddle, C., Malek, M., Sharp, W., et al. (2011). Cortical development in typically developing children with symptoms of hyperactivity and impulsivity: Support for a dimensional view of attention deficit hyperactivity disorder. *American Journal of Psychiatry, 168*(2), 143–151.

Sheslow, D., & Adams, W. (2003). *Wide Range Assessment of Memory and Learning–Revised (WRAML-2): Administration and technical manual.* Lutz, FL: Psychological Assessment Resources.

Siegel, L. (2013). *Understanding dyslexia and other learning disabilities.* Vancouver, Canada: Pacific Educational Press.

Siegel, L. S., & Ryan, E. B. (1989). The development of working memory in normally achieving and subtypes of learning disabled children. *Child Development, 60,* 973–980.

Snodgrass, J. G., & Vanderwart, M. (1980). A standardized set of 260 pictures: Norms for name agreement, image agreement, familiarity, and visual complexity. *Journal of Experimental Psychology: Human Learning and Memory, 6*(2), 174.

Snowling, M. J. (1996). Dyslexia: A hundred years on. *British Medical Journal, 313*(7065), 1096.

Solodow, W., Sandy, S. V., Leventhal, F., Beszylko, S., Shepherd, M. J., Cohen, J., et al. (2006). Frequency and diagnostic criteria for nonverbal learning disabilities in a general learning disability school cohort. *Thalamus, 24,* 17–33.

Soma, Y., Nakamura, K., Oyama, M., Tsuchiya, Y., & Yamamoto, M. (2009). Prevalence of attention-deficit/hyperactivity disorder (ADHD) symptoms in preschool children: Discrepancy between parent and teacher evaluations. *Environmental Health and Preventive Medicine, 14*(2), 150–154.

Spelke, E., Lee, S. A., & Izard, V. (2010). Beyond core knowledge: Natural geometry. *Cognitive Science, 34*(5), 863–884.

Spinnler, H., & Tognoni, G. (1987). Taratura e standardizzazione di test neuropsicologici [Standardization of neuropsychological tests]. *Italian Journal of Neurosciences, 8,* 35–38.

Spreen, O. (2011). Nonverbal learning disabilities: A critical review. *Child Neuropsychology, 17,* 418–443.

Stambak, M. (1951). Le problème du rythme dans le développement de l'enfant et dans les dyslexies d'évolution. *Enfance, 4,* 480–502.

Stanfield, A. C., McIntosh, A. M., Spencer, M. D., Philip, R., Gaur, S., & Lawrie, S. M. (2008). Towards a neuroanatomy of autism: A systematic review and meta-analysis of structural magnetic resonance imaging studies. *European Psychiatry, 23*(4), 289–299.

Staniloiu, A., & Markowitsch, H. J. (2012). A rapprochement between emotion and cognition: Amygdala, emotion, and self-relevance in episodic-autobiographical memory. *Behavioral and Brain Sciences, 35*(3), 164–166.

Stiles, J., Appelbaum, M., Nass, R., & Trauner, D. (2008). Effects of early focal brain injury on memory for visuospatial patterns: Selective deficits of global–local processing. *Neuropsychology, 22,* 61–73.

Stiles-Davis, J., Janowsky, J., Engel, M., & Nass, R. (1988). Drawing ability in four young children with congenital unilateral brain lesions. *Neuropsychologia, 26*(3), 359–371.

Strang, J. D., & Rourke, B. P. (1983). Concept-formation/non-verbal reasoning abilities of children who exhibit specific academic problems with arithmetic. *Journal of Clinical Child and Adolescent Psychology, 12*(1), 33–39.

Strang, J. D., & Rourke, B. P. (1985). Arithmetic disability subtypes: The neuropsychological significance of specific arithmetical impairment in childhood. In B. P. Rourke (Ed.), *Neuropsychology of learning disabilities: Essentials of subtype analysis* (pp. 167–183). New York: Guilford Press.

Strauss, A. A., & Lehtinen, L. E. (1947). *Psychopathology and education of the brain-injured child.* New York: Grune & Stratton.

Swillen, A., Vandeputte, L., Cracco, J., Maes, B., Ghesquière, P., Devriendt, K., et al. (1999). Neuropsychological, learning and psychosocial profile of primary school aged children with the velo–cardio–facial syndrome (22q11 deletion): Evidence for a nonverbal learning disability? *Child Neuropsychology, 5*(4), 230–241.

Szucs, D., Devine, A., Soltesz, F., Nobes, A., & Gabriel, F. (2013). Developmental dyscalculia is related to visuo–spatial memory and inhibition impairment. *Cortex, 49*(10), 2674–2688.

Tanguay, P. (2001). *Nonverbal learning disabilities at home: A parent's guide.* London: Jessica Kingsley.

Telzrow, C. E., & Bonar, A. M. (2001). Responding to students with nonverbal learning disabilities. *Teaching Exceptional Children, 34*, 8–13.

Ternes, J., Woody, R., & Livingston, R. (1987). Case report: A child with right hemisphere deficit syndrome responsive to carbamazepine treatment. *Journal of the American Academy of Child and Adolescent Psychiatry, 26*(4), 586–588.

Thompson, S. J., Auslander, W. F., & White, N. H. (2001). Comparison of single-mother and two-parent families on metabolic control of children with diabetes. *Diabetes Care, 24*(2), 234–238.

Thurstone, L. L., & Thurstone, T. G. (1963). *Primary mental abilities.* Chicago: Science Research Associates.

Tiffin, J. (1968). *Purdue Pegboard: Examiner manual.* Chicago: Science Research Associates.

Torgesen, J. K., Wagner, R., & Rashotte, C. (1999). *TOWRE–2 Test of Word Reading Efficiency.* Austin, TX: PRO-ED.

Tranel, D., Hall, L. E., Olson, S., & Tranel, N. N. (1987). Evidence for a right hemisphere developmental learning disability. *Developmental Neuropsychology, 3*, 113–127.

Tressoldi, P. E., & Cornoldi, C. (1991). *Batteria per la valutazione della scrittura e della competenza ortografica nella scuola dell'obbligo.* Florence, Italy: Giunti O.S.-Organizzazioni Speciali.

Tressoldi, P. E., Cornoldi, C., & Re, A. M. (2012). *BVSCO-2: Batteria per la Valutazione della Scrittura e della Competenza Ortografica-2.* Florence, Italy: Giunti O.S.-Organizzazioni Speciali.

Tsatsanis, K. D., Fuerst, D. R., & Rourke, B. P. (1997). Psychosocial dimensions of learning disabilities: External validation and relationship with age and academic functioning. *Journal of Learning Disabilities, 30*(5), 490–502.

Tsatsanis, K. D., & Rourke, B. P. (2003). Syndrome of nonverbal learning disabilities: Effects on learning. In A. Fine & R. Kotkin (Eds.), *Therapist's guide to learning and attention disorders* (pp. 109–145). Cambridge, MA: Academic Press.

Tunali, B., & Power, T. G. (1993). Creating satisfaction: A psychological perspective on stress and coping in families of handicapped children. *Journal of Child Psychology and Psychiatry, 34*(6), 945–957.

Van Luit, J. E. (2009). Nonverbal learning disabilities and arithmetic problems: The effectiveness of an explicit verbal instruction model. *Advances in Learning and Behavioral Disabilities, 22*, 265–289.

Varnhagen, C. K., Lewin, S., Das, J. P., Bowen, P., Ma, K., & Klimek, M. (1988). Neurofibromatosis and psychological processes. *Journal of Developmental and Behavioral Pediatrics, 9*(5), 257–265.

Vecchi, T., & Richardson, T. E. (2000). Active processing in visuo–spatial working memory. *Cahiers de Psychologie Cognitive, 19*, 3–32.

Venneri, A., Cornoldi, C., & Garuti, M. (2003). Arithmetic difficulties in children with visuospatial learning disability (VLD). *Child Neuropsychology, 9*(3), 175–183.

Vernon, P. (1964). *The structure of human abilities.* London: Methuen.

Vicari, S., Caravale, B., Carlesimo, G. A., Casadei, A. M., & Allemand, F. (2004). Spatial working memory deficits in children at ages 3–4 who were low birth weight, preterm infants. *Neuropsychology, 18*, 673–678.

Vicari, S., Stiles, J., Stern, C., & Resca, A. (1998). Spatial grouping activity in children with early cortical and subcortical lesions. *Developmental Medicine and Child Neurology, 40*(2), 90–99.

Voeller, K. K. (1986). Right-hemisphere deficit syndrome in children. *American Journal of Psychiatry, 143*(8), 1004–1009.

Walton, G. M., & Cohen, G. L. (2007). A question of belonging: Race, social fit, and achievement. *Journal of Personality and Social Psychology, 92*(1), 82.

Walton, G. M., & Cohen, G. L. (2011). A brief social-belonging intervention improves academic and health outcomes of minority students. *Science, 331*(6023), 1447–1451.

Warren, R. (2003). Drawing on the wrong side of the brain: An art teacher's case for recognising NLD. *International Journal of Art and Design Education, 22*(3), 325–334.

Webster-Stratton, C. (1990). Stress: A potential disruptor of parent perceptions and family interactions. *Journal of Clinical Child Psychology, 19*(4), 302–312.

Wechsler, D. (1949). *Wechsler Intelligence Scale for Children manual.* New York: Psychological Corp.

Wechsler, D. (1974). *Manual for the Wechsler Intelligence Scale for Children–Revised.* New York: Psychological Corp.

Wechsler, D. (1991). *Wechsler Intelligence Scale for Children–Third Edition.* San Antonio, TX: Psychological Corp.

Wechsler, D. (1999). *Wechsler Abbreviated Scale of Intelligence (WASI).* Bloomington, MN: Pearson.

Wechsler, D. (2003). *Wechsler Intelligence Scale for Children–Fourth Edition.* San Antonio, TX: Psychological Corp.

Wechsler, D. (2014). *Wechsler Intelligence Scale for Children–Fifth Edition*. Bloomington, MN: Pearson.

Weintraub, S., & Mesulam, M. M. (1983). Developmental learning disabilities of the right hemisphere: Emotional, interpersonal, and cognitive components. *Archives of Neurology, 40*(8), 463–468.

Weyandt, L., Swentosky, A., & Gudmundsdottir, B. G. (2013). Neuroimaging and ADHD: fMRI, PET, DTI findings, and methodological limitations. *Developmental Neuropsychology, 38*(4), 211–225.

Wiederholt, J. L., & Bryant, B. R. (2012). *Gray Oral Reading Tests–Fifth Edition (GORT-5)*. Austin, TX: PRO-ED.

Wilkinson, G. S., & Robertson, G. J. (2006). *Wide Range Achievement Test– Fourth Edition*. Lutz, FL: Psychological Assessment Resources.

Wilson, B. N., Kaplan, B. J., Crawford, S. G., & Roberts, G. (2007). *The Developmental Coordination Disorder Questionnaire 2007 DCDQ'07*. Alberta, Canada: Alberta Children's Hospital.

Wirt, R. D., Lachar, D., Klinedinst, J. K., & Seat, P. D. (1977). *Multidimensional description of child personality: A manual for the Personality Inventory for Children*. Los Angeles: Western Psychological Services.

Woodcock, R. W., McGrew, K. S., & Mather, N. (2001). *Woodcock–Johnson® III NU Tests of Achievement*. Rolling Meadows, IL: Riverside.

Woodcock, R. W., McGrew, K. S., & Mather, N. (2007). *Woodcock–Johnson® III Diagnostic supplement to the tests of cognitive abilities*. Rolling Meadows, IL: Riverside.

World Health Organization. (1992). *International classification of diseases and related disorders (ICD-10)*. Geneva, Switzerland: Author.

Worling, D. E., Humphries, T., & Tannock, R. (1999). Spatial and emotional aspects of language inferencing in nonverbal learning disabilities. *Brain and Language, 70*(2), 220–239.

Youngstrom, E., Loeber, R., & Stouthamer-Loeber, M. (2000). Patterns and correlates of agreement between parent, teacher, and male adolescent ratings of externalizing and internalizing problems. *Journal of Consulting and Clinical Psychology, 68*(6), 1038.

Yu, J., Buka, S., McCormick, M. C., Fitzmaurice, G. M., & Indurkhya, A. (2006). Behavioral problems and the effects of early intervention on eight-year-old children with learning disabilities. *Maternal and Child Health Journal, 10*, 329–338.

Zazzo, R. (1951). Un travail d'équipe: Réflexions à propos du symposium sur les dyslexies. *Enfance, 4*(5), 385–388.

Index

Note: *f* following a page number indicates a figure; *t* indicates a table.